PENGUIN BOOKS

WISH I COULD BE THERE

Allen Shawn is a composer and writer. He began composing music at the age of ten and has produced a large catalog of orchestral, chamber, vocal, and piano works, as well as music for ballet, theater, and film. He performs frequently as a pianist. His previous book is *Arnold Schoenberg's Journey*, and he has also written for the *Atlantic Monthly*. He is on the faculty at Bennington College and lives in Vermont.

Natural selection is the guiding agent of evolution, but it is not an all-seeing and all-wise pilot. It adapts, as best it can, a living species to the environments prevailing in a given place at a given time, but it cannot know the future.

—Theodosius Dobzhansky, *Evolution*

They cannot scare me with their empty spaces
Between stars—on stars where no human race is.
I have it in me so much nearer home
To scare myself with my own desert places.

—Robert Frost, "Desert Places"

Foreword

I am a composer, pianist, and teacher. My previous book was about the great Austrian composer Arnold Schoenberg.

Four years ago a close friend of mine suggested that I write a book about my phobias. "After all you are an expert," he said. I was taken aback by his suggestion, voicing my resistance logically, answering that I was not an expert, but simply a sufferer. "Therein lies your expertise," he replied. "And be sure to emphasize in your book to what degree your phobias have harmed your life," he added, helpfully.

It always hurts to hear one's defects and difficulties referred to by others simply as facts. I wanted to wriggle out of his suggestion and even out of his description of me as an expert in phobias through suffering, to detach myself from my handicap as if my personality and my strengths belonged to one person, my problems to another. While my agoraphobia has plagued me my entire adult life, I balked at the idea of presenting this aspect of myself in print. The topic is a dark one, reflecting a side of my life I can normally escape from in my creative work. And, despite my love of investigation, I shrank from delving into a subject requiring a type and degree of learning I do not possess.

Nevertheless, I soon embarked on this project, as if it were my fate to do so. Ultimately it led me on a search that was not only fascinating, but actually life changing. The search was both internal, into my own personal past, and external, into regions of science and psychology which required every ounce of mental acuity I could muster. The result is the book you hold in your hands.

To write about one's own difficulties and their possible origins is not a task that lends itself to clear conclusions. The very nature of these difficulties and limitations is slippery. How can I know that, now that I have written about myself, the reader will conclude that my problems can even be summarized as phobias? I cannot. Who can truly see himself analytically, and with clarity? Furthermore, it is surely unknowable how much of who we are as adults is determined by impersonal factors, such as our genetic makeup, and how much by experiences unique to us as individuals, our childhood environment, chance events that have occurred to us, the choices we ourselves have made along the way. Therefore, I have interwoven two distinctly different ways of approaching my subject. I have written about my own childhood as I remember it, from within, and about the subjects I investigated—the brain, the physiology of fear, the way we form habits of thought and behavior, what Freud was trying to describe of the inner life of the mind—as I understood them, as a layman trying to grasp the origins, both personal and universal, of his own predicament. It would be tiresome to reiterate at each juncture along the way that I am not a biologist, neurologist, or psychologist, and that this is not a conventional memoir, so I remind the reader of these facts only occasionally.

This book is not about cure, and it offers no certainties. Its structure is that of a spiral, or, if you prefer, like the overlapping, connected folds of a brain. While the subject of phobias was my point of departure, I believe that this book is actually about a search for understanding the origins of the quirks of personality we all have, the flaws inherent in being human.

I come from a literary family. My father was William Shawn, editor of *The New Yorker* magazine for thirty-five years, and my brother is Wallace Shawn, the playwright and actor. My mother was Cecille Lyon Shawn, who had a career as a journalist and editor when she was in her twenties. My twin sister, Mary, is mentally retarded and lives in an institution in Delaware. In the autobiographical portions of the book, I have tried to convey the flavor of my childhood world, but I have also kept my focus on the possible sources of my own psychological handicaps and have not attempted a memoir in a more comprehensive sense. For many years I was married. I have not dealt with that period of my life in this book, nor have I written about my children, Annie and Harold, who belong to the joyful and fulfilling aspects of my life which are, by and large, not my focus here. By not using names in the autobiographical portions of the book— except in the case of my sister—I have deliberately tried to make my own past into something of an abstraction so that the reader is encouraged to think about his or her own life. What is told is true, but it is an incomplete account. Indeed, most people who know me may not even recognize the self I describe here. As a self-portrait, it is a bit like a photo cropped so that only my shadow is visible. Yet, regrettably, this is a shadow that accompanies me everywhere, indoors and out, in all weather, and probably always will.

In writing the book I came to the conclusion that the shame I originally felt at the prospect of writing it was a fear worth conquering. My hunch is that beneath the surface of even the most smoothly functioning lives (and families) there are always fissures— psychological crises, deficits, conflicts. By putting my own worst foot forward, as it were, I mean to challenge our assumptions about what a normal person is.

Many people and many books have aided me in my search. I have tried to acknowledge them at the end of the book. Although I have checked my facts, I speak here only from a layman's perspective. For those who recognize themselves in this book, I hope that it can provide useful information, as well as the pleasure of seeing inner experiences articulated. For those who recognize a friend or lover or parent or child in this account, I hope it is a source of understanding.

Contents

Introduction

I am driving down a dirt road in the woods to a friend's house. He didn't say how many miles down his house was. He did say it was beautiful there, on the lake, so I had suggested to E that she come along, and she is sitting next to me, chatting. The car jerks and bucks on the rut-filled path. There aren't any houses in view. I start looking for mailboxes and don't see any. I can't see any driveways leading to concealed houses either. It would appear that the road is quite isolated.

I am fine for the first mile but slowly start to feel as if I were suffocating. The woods are dense, and all I can see are trees. Occasionally a branch strikes the windshield. I feel as if I need to find a bathroom. My breaths are becoming short and shallow, and a dark cloud seems to be forming in front of my eyes. I keep looking for houses, and there aren't any. Without noticing it, I slip into a dreamlike state, wherein the passage of time has slowed painfully, as if I have been driving down the road for hours. My eyes are straining through a dark, blurry film. I feel as if I were floating, as if I were only partly in my own body, only partly still in the car. E is still cheerfully speaking but sounds both irritating and distant, as if we were separated by an invisible screen through which her usually melodious voice sounds grating. I say a few words in response that come out sounding pinched, curt, and crabby.

The odometer says we have been driving for four and a half

miles, but the numbers have no meaning. I am growing confused and resentful and agitated. The road back will be bumpy
and slow too, I think, and wasn't there a fork back there at some
point that I have already taken? How will I remember the way
back? My legs are stiff and heavy, and I am trembling. I want to
turn the car around. The road seems to grow darker. My muscles
are coiled around one another, pulled taut. I am breaking, more
and more confused, and I can't breathe. There's no sky overhead.

I turn the car around.

I'm working on this "agoraphobia" problem. I started going for
treatment again about a year and a half ago. It is my third serious
effort to do so. I am fifty-seven years old, but tackling this problem again makes me feel as if I were five. In the course of this
work I have made a little progress and have gained some new
perspectives on the condition. In a sense it is a trivial problem,
merely an inconvenient personality trait. It can't be compared for
a moment with suffering a life-threatening illness, being caught
in a war, being subject to injustice and persecution, or countless
other torments that people face all over the world. I would even
surmise that serious adversity might, as it were, interrupt such a
neurotic symptom. But as I have worked on the problem, I have
also found it more and more intriguing.

One might speculate that a boy who grew up in the woods
probably wouldn't have a woods phobia. But life isn't that simple. I grew up in New York City, where I ultimately acquired a
number of urban fears, and in some ways being in the country
allows me to escape from them.

I now live in Vermont and routinely travel to New York,
New Jersey, Massachusetts, parts of New Hampshire, and Con-
necticut. I stay not only within the radius of five states but also

within a clearly practiced itinerary. I always take the same roads, what most people call the service roads. I won't drive on highways unless there are frequent exits and visible towns along the way. Recently I went south of New York for the first time in fifteen years. I last flew (to La Jolla, California) in the summer of 1993. Even though I was medicated, my teeth chattered for the entire trip, and I didn't experience a hoped-for breakthrough, a revelation that flying was easy. Admittedly I was amazed while on the plane by how routine it was. I remember thinking: "I get it! It's just a bus that happens to be up in the air." But once I was on the ground again, the old dread returned in full force. Even being on a plane on the runway with the door shut is a dreadful prospect to me.

Driving from where I live in Vermont to New York City doesn't particularly bother me, but before doing the four-hour evening drive (I prefer the evening because there is less traffic), I am sad, jittery, and slightly irritable all day, grimly going through the motions of life. Sometimes I end up with a heavy, bulging suitcase even if the trip will only be for twenty-four hours. Instead of packing one tie, I pack six or seven, to have more options. By the time the evening comes around, I have repeatedly checked what I am bringing and have added pads of paper, or books, or recordings I just might need but probably won't. The depression, if that's what it is, feels more and more external, like a fact about the world. It is as if I were about to undergo surgery or worse. It becomes difficult to focus on any but the most mundane tasks. My thoughts flicker haphazardly like moths around lamps, unable to settle anywhere. It is possible to wash dishes alongside this mental static, but not to read. The idea of the long drive gets mixed up with feelings of loss and guilt, thoughts of other journeys, and moments long forgotten that, in memory, are tinged with sadness. I think of seeing my father waving and

crying and sliding to the left through the grimy windows of the
train pulling me out of Grand Central Station on the way to
music camp; of my sister in a party dress on a swing in Chatham,
Massachusetts; of my mother, sitting next to me in a dark, air-
conditioned movie theater on an unexpected outing in mid-
summer.

Some form of this same downcast, nervous mental state is a
universal part of the phobic process. It is called anticipatory
anxiety, and apparently, as one recovers from phobias (if one
does), it is the slowest phobic symptom to disappear.

Were I now to unfold for you a scroll upon which I had
written my phobias, it might stretch all the way to China. I don't
like heights. I don't like being on the water. I am upset by walking across parking lots or open parks or fields where there are no
buildings. I tend to avoid bridges, unless they are on a small scale.
I respond poorly to stretches of vastness but do equally badly
when I am closed in, as I am severely claustrophobic. When I go
to a theater, I sit on the aisle. I am petrified of tunnels, making
most train travel as well as many drives difficult. I don't take
subways. I avoid elevators as much as possible. I experience
glassed-in spaces as toxic, and I find it very difficult to adjust to
being in buildings in which the windows don't open. I don't like
to go to enclosed malls; and if I do, I don't venture very far into
them. Even large museums cause me problems, despite my hunger
to visit them. In short, I am afraid both of closed and of open
spaces, and I am afraid, in a sense, of any form of isolation. When
I am invited to a new house or apartment or to an event of any
kind, my first reaction is to worry about its location. Often I go.
But I end up missing things and harming or losing relationships.
When I am in settings that are far from my own home, I sometimes do adjust. But just as often my body lapses into a kind of

closed hypervigilance or maintains a steady interior tremor like a car engine stalled in traffic.

The degree of my self-preoccupation is appalling.

Occasionally I gear myself up for a new trip. Over the past twenty years I have traveled by train to Atlanta, Rochester, New York, Ithaca, and Washington, D.C.; by car to Montreal (for an hour); and, in 1990, by boat to France, where I once lived for two years. But each excursion is an isolated accomplishment that doesn't particularly change my character overall. In each case I am almost frozen with anticipatory anxiety for weeks or months in advance and am exhausted, if pleased, afterward. Often these trips are more than worth it, for myself and for others. But overall, progress is slow. Fortunately, by chipping away at the various roads in my part of the country, I am now familiar with enough places to be able to move around contentedly. But it is within a circumscribed world and without spontaneity.

Behind every arrival at a new destination lies a series of test runs, many of which are failures. A recent trip to Syracuse, New York, to hear the orchestra there play one of my pieces, required no less than six attempted trips in advance, as I repeatedly rejected routes as intolerable, returning to a point of reference that I came to know well. In an effort to keep myself together while on the road, I develop a rather compulsive connection to such spots along the way, not unlike the way my mother used to keep Mr. Paine, the shoe salesman, or Joe, the butcher, in her sights, as if they were solid steel posts of reliability in a dangerous world. Along the way to Syracuse a McDonald's decorated in fifties diner style became a secure foothold for me. When I returned to it and heard the jukebox playing "Great Balls of Fire" and saw the life-size plastic statue of Elvis and the posters of Mick Jagger, I would breathe more easily. In the men's room was a framed poster of five torso-length portraits of the young Marilyn Monroe, five breezy, completely unforced poses. In the pictures she wore a white sweater and a necklace of alternating amber and black oval stones. The thought that she had long ago been chemically reabsorbed into the earth did not detract from the comforting power of her smiling, relaxed gaze.

All this would be funny were it not sad. Even I myself laugh thinking about it and forget the pain, the fact that behind each of these self-imposed restrictions lie experiences of intense anguish. I tend not to talk about the subject. We all have "problems," after all. The women in my life have lived with this firsthand and tried to put up with it, as have my wonderful children, but even my own brother and most of my friends don't know more about it than that I tend to avoid certain experiences.

What precisely is the matter?

A part of me wishes to turn away from the topic or at least to describe it in the third person. But that abhorrence is actually part of the problem. I reassure myself that my readers are all human and that to be human is to experience limitations of many kinds. Besides, at those moments when we are in the grip of an inner force, perhaps something important is being revealed.

Chapter One

Demons on My Back

The mind is its own place and in itself
Can make a heav'n of hell, A hell of heav'n.
—John Milton

In the mid-1970s I was in my late twenties and living on New York's Upper West Side with my French girlfriend, teaching music at three schools to earn a living. One Halloween night I was returning home to my apartment building in my beige, imitation camel-hair overcoat, carrying some packages from the supermarket. I had gotten through the door of the small vestibule next to the apartment buzzers and was awkwardly fumbling for my keys to the inner door while holding the groceries against it when three boys crashed through the entrance behind me and jumped on top of me. In an instant they were holding me down and demanding money. I was trapped. "Take my coat! Take my coat!" I yelled breathlessly, allowing it to be peeled off me. (I didn't have much money, and the coat was one of my prized possessions.) I can still remember the strength with which I tried to throw the attackers off my back. As I struggled, an image came into my mind of a huge prehistoric animal with an enormous hard shell beneath its shoulders, a back that could carry enormous weight and throw off heavy beasts. I am in fact a small man, but I remember that my efforts against the would-be thieves were not completely futile. I was fierce. Still, it was fortunate that a neighbor on the first floor heard the commotion, opened his apartment door, and yelled, scattering my tormentors. Suddenly the tiny space I had been trapped in was once again a benign entranceway. A soothing autumn breeze blew through the open door.

Only gradually—as I tremulously picked up the fallen groceries and my discarded coat (now with a ripped sleeve) and slowly made my way to the elevator, trying to resume breathing normally and to quiet my racing heart—did it occur to me that I might have just narrowly escaped being badly hurt or even killed.

As I rode the elevator, I thought of the strength that I had felt, and I tried to remember what had gone through my mind, something like "I've got to get them off me; I've got to get them off me." Nobody likes being mugged. Then I realized that what had made me summon up all my strength in the vestibule was not the threat of being robbed or the threat of death or that of being hurt, but the fact that I was being *held down*. My lifelong claustrophobia had awakened in me an intensity of physical response that the realistic danger of being harmed might not have. In the face of my Halloween attackers I *was* afraid, but no more afraid than the next person would be. However, I was phobic about being held down, and this brought out every ounce of strength I had within me. As I thought all this, the elevator doors opened, and I realized that I had been holding my breath since

I'd stepped inside. I exhaled with relief and headed toward my apartment to tell my girlfriend what had happened.

Similar as they look and feel, fear and phobia are not the same. Yet the line between them is often hard to delineate. Indeed they can be experienced simultaneously.

The fact that an animal image came to my mind as I tried to heave my attackers off me that Halloween night was of course not a coincidence. When we are afraid, we experience the surge of adrenaline associated with the well-known fight-or-flight syndrome, part of the automatic defense response humans share with most living creatures. Beneath our fearful thoughts is an ancient systemic process. In purely phobic reactions, this same physiological response, which in emergencies readies an animal or a human to respond with extra alertness, speed, strength, and effectiveness to a threat, is triggered seemingly haphazardly by situations or objects that in fact pose no actual or immediate danger. When the same responses one might feel being suddenly attacked occur in reaction to an apparently innocuous circumstance—such as a walk across a large open parking lot or an elevator ride or lunch in a restaurant—the physical symptoms make no rational sense and therefore become a crisis on their own account.

Under such conditions the mind races to pin a logical explanation on the body's panic. A sudden rapid heartbeat, pain in the chest, flushing of the face, queasiness in the stomach, blurring of vision, tingling and coldness in the hands, the sensation of choking, shortness of breath, tension in the limbs—these symptoms can only signal to the brain that the organism it monitors must be in danger. After all, failing an organic cause, these responses are associated with self-protection; why else would they be mobilized if there were nothing to be protected from? Unable to determine an extrinsic emergency, the mind turns inward to explain the threat, manufacturing logical conclusions: One is in physical or mental crisis. There ensues a kind of distancing effect, a physiologically triggered impression of unreality. One sees oneself as if from outside, while coping with the mental confusion and spiraling fearful thoughts that also come with the body's responses and that in turn further the physical symptoms.

While the body is primed to respond to an emergency, it is not primed to swiftly send out an all-clear signal once the emergency response is in full throttle. In situations of true danger, after all, additional vigilance may be advisable. Nature has thus provided that the chemical processes of fear not only initiate quickly but also subside gradually, like one of those sirens that reach a high peak in a few seconds and then slowly, evenly descend to their lowest tones. Therefore, although panic declines surprisingly quickly on its own, it leaves a chemical residue that makes one feel strangely irritable and tired.

What makes the phobic person unusually susceptible to triggers to the anxiety cycle is a matter for debate; explanations continue to evolve. Heredity—chemical predisposition—is strongly indicated. Upbringing is an undeniable factor. Imitation of a phobic parent is almost universally present.

But why a phobia of this and not of that? Why does the man who dreads public speaking love to fly his own plane? Why does the woman who is appearing on the talk show dread the elevator in the building but not her appearance on the show itself? Although a phobia can sometimes be the result of one bad experience or influence, its origins are often mysterious. To discuss phobias takes us both into the realm of physiology and into the realm of personal history, where traumatic experiences, modeling (fears inculcated by observing role models), and the importance of symbolism all may come into play.

One thing is clear: to describe the reaction simply as a mental phenomenon is misleading. By the time it constitutes a "problem," it has become a habitual response of both body and mind, as automatic as an allergic reaction and equally impervious to willpower. I myself am as able to cope with normal nervousness as the next person. I know what it is to be anxious before performing in a concert or giving a talk, being interviewed for a job, or anticipating a painful confrontation with a colleague or friend. I know what it is to take a deep breath before such occasions and face them. But even after many years of effort I have not conquered my phobia. People have known for centuries how entrenched phobias can become. As early as 1621 Robert Burton, in his *Anatomy of Melancholy,* pointed out that phobic terror (though not as yet identified by that term) was immune to normal reasoning: "[c]ounsel can do little good: you may as well bid him that . . . is wounded, not to feel pain."

The phobic person is gripped by specific dreads, of objects or situations, even while the phobias of others appear to him irrational. But whatever the object of the phobia, in every case the physical and psychological responses are drawn from the same bodily repertoire. From an objective point of view, then, it is clearly the phobic reaction itself, not the dreaded object or situation, that is the culprit. However, we do not live our lives objectively. If you bang your head against a door, and someone tells you that the door was "only in your imagination," you're going to respond that whatever it was, it hurt. Like pain, fear is a sign, a sign that something is wrong. A phobia is like a pain in the soul.

The word *phobia* comes from the Greek word for fear, *phobos.* It was first used in the first century by the Roman encyclopedist Celsus, who invented the term "hydrophobia" to connote the fear of water. By borrowing the word for fear, Celsus clearly sought to convey the fact that a phobia has all the characteristics of fear. It looks and feels like fear and makes one behave as one does when afraid. Yet it also seems, to the rational mind, either out of proportion to any possible danger (taking a swim does not ensure drowning) or entirely misplaced (going near water is normally not dangerous). From Celsus spread the idea of attaching the suffix "phobia" to any object eliciting such irrational dread. From a diagnostic point of view, *phobia* is now considered "persistent and irrational fear of any specific object, activity, or situation that results in a compelling desire to avoid the feared or phobic stimulus."

The paramount characteristics of fear are a heightened vigilance—the sense of being on high alert—and the compulsion to flee what is feared. The reaction in phobia is identical. One friend in her twenties told me that she believed that her fear of spiders dated from an incident when she was eight years old. Her brother tricked her into walking under a spiderweb, and the spider had landed on her head. These days, if she sees a spider in her bedroom, she cannot go to sleep unless she is certain the spider has been killed or taken away. Another friend, R, takes to her heels if a mouse is in her house and waits outside until a member of her family has dealt with it. She describes the mouse as occupying "her entire mind" at such moments. My friend P describes her response to moths similarly: "I used to have a huge fear of moths. Strange, isn't it? I would flee a room if a tiny moth was present. I could be in the middle of a meeting, it didn't matter, I would just get up and leave. I don't do that now, but I still feel it. It's a very physical thing, that fear. But now I can make myself stay, and I can even trap the moth (in a yogurt container or jar) and let it out of the house. This took me years. I'm not paralyzed by it now, thankfully. It's partly because R helped me really look at them and helped me relax and see what they really are like. It took some degree of patience on his part. What's strange about it is that I never feared butterflies."

Discrete phobias (airplanes, bridges, tunnels, open spaces, spiders, etc.) are commonly referred to as specific phobias. Such phobias truly run the gamut and are by no means confined to likely objects of revulsion. It is as surprising how common many specific phobias are, a sign that they are indeed rooted in universal responses, as it is how very specific and nuanced they can be. A phobia of mice and rats is common, but one of squirrels, a rodent with a tail, much less so. Small, furry creatures with wings, bats, disturb many more people than do birds. In fact ornithophobia is rather rare. All those who fear flying do not have the same reasons. In some claustrophobia is the central issue; in others it may be the social aspects of the experience; in still others it is the fear of the plane's crashing. A fear of elevators is common. But even this fear can be broken down further into myriad subcategories; the degree of dread can vary according to whether the elevators have or do not have windows, are made of metal or of wood, have or do not have piped-in Muzak, are automated or are manually operated, etc. My father, who avoided most elevators, was almost comfortable in an elevator that was manually operated.

These days specific phobias of objects and physical surroundings are distinguished from the social phobias, fears that involve such situations as public speaking and eating in public, in which one will be subject to "scrutiny by others." Sometimes the specific phobia category is further broken down into subcategories:

1. Fears of animals
2. Fears of some aspect of the natural environment (heights, thunder, etc.)
3. Fears of situations (elevators, tunnels, etc.)

4. Miscellaneous fears not covered above (germs, noise)
5. Fears of blood, injection, or injury or references to these

This last type has the distinction of being associated with the physical reaction of fainting. Contrary to the evidence provided in many a silent film and cartoon, in which people faint dead away when confronted with danger or shock, in most circumstances in which phobia sufferers may be afraid of fainting or even feel faint, the elevated blood pressure that accompanies their phobic response actually prevents this from happening. The so-called blood-injury-injection response alone slows the heart rate and lowers the blood pressure, a requisite for loss of consciousness. But the blood and injury phobia *can* overlap with other categories, of course—with fears of animals, say, or with the claustrophobic dread of being in a dentist's chair. In addition, all specific phobias can overlap with social phobias in that they cause changes in behavior or avoidances that either engender shame or are motivated by it.

There is an additional view that the notion of disgust is a more prevalent emotional component in some phobias than fear. Disgust phobias include aversions to such creatures as insects, worms, and slugs, for example, or the phobia of disorder or of germs.

The specific phobia category, while convenient in terms of developing broadly applicable treatments, glosses over important distinctions. Those common fears that would appear to be of a quasi-instinctual kind, having a connection to—or roots in—realistic dangers (fear of the dark, of water, of confinement, of potentially dangerous animals), should surely be distinguished from those far rarer ones that could probably be acquired only by highly personal association and experiences (fear of clowns, of speaking on the telephone, of moths, of buttons). While one might be able to approach the problem of a fear of water primarily with some kind of progressive desensitization, one would surely need to talk about the clowns.

A phobia in the latter category troubled an early patient of Freud's, a man who felt an ungovernable terror when he saw anyone wearing a mask. The patient told Freud that he had a particular horror of a mask's "fixity" of expression. Freud postulated that a traumatic childhood experience lay behind this fear. Eventually he uncovered that at the age of three the patient had in fact been left alone with the body of his dead mother as she lay in bed, awaiting burial. The patient had no memory of this childhood trauma, but it was authenticated by his older sister. The immobility he feared seeing in a mask was something he had once confronted in his dead mother's immobile face. Learning this cured the patient of his phobia by disentangling the impact of his devastating original life crisis from the benign objects that mimicked it.

Some phobic triggers cause a revulsion even in a picture or as a passing reference in a conversation, and others are distressing only when actually encountered. Those who dread being on an airplane don't mind seeing one in a picture. Some phobias have connections to very real physical sensations—for example, those induced by looking up or down to a great height. It is not the "view" from the top of a mountain that frightens one who "fears" heights, but the experience of looking down. Other phobias may have their ties to minor physical ailments affecting vision, hearing, breathing, and balance.

In fact the world of phobias is vast. In the course of working on this book I have often found myself questioning if we are not lumping a number of distinctly different phenomena into this one category. The concept of phobia encompasses a whole range of social dreads, including stage fright; the fear of public speaking, eating in public, being looked at (scopophobia); fears of creatures: dogs, cats, frogs, insects, snakes, birds, spiders, even fish; fears of height (acrophobia) and depth (bathophobia); fears of confinement; fears of being in the open; fears of being in the forest; fears of being indoors. There are weather phobias— fear of thunder, rainstorms (ombrophobia), snow, lightning. One can have a phobia of drafts or of moisture. One can have a phobia of stars (siderophobia). There are those who have a morbid fear of nakedness (gymnophobia) or of sex (genophobia), and those who fear pleasure (hedonophobia). There is a phobia of disorder or untidiness (ataxophobia). Some people have a fear of the sound of their own voices (phonophobia) or of seeing themselves in a mirror (eisotrophobia). There is a phobia of standing (stasiphobia), and of walking; there is a phobia of sitting down (thaasophobia). There are fears that come close to being simply a fear of being on this earth: the fear of light (photophobia), of air (aerophobia). Most circularly of all, there is the phobia of acquiring phobias (phobophobia).

Phobias can spread from specificity (being shut in a laundry closet) to generalization (all confinement, of every kind) but can also remain remarkably individualized. In recent days I have read of a tennis player who had a dread of fuzzy things and therefore wore gloves when he played; of someone who avoided all brown objects and could not move toward anything of that color; of a woman who had a severe phobia of chicken legs. Every time she was asked to a party she had to call up and ask, "You're not serving chicken legs, are you?" The one time she went to a party and there were chicken parts for dinner, she had a huge reaction. She had to be taken to the emergency room. The actor Richard Burton could not remain in a room with a jar of honey, even if it was concealed in a drawer. These rare phobias come close to constituting what we might call superstitions. Yet their impact on daily life is surprisingly deep. In other cases more common phobias are taken to extraordinary lengths. One woman could not bathe her child or take a normal bath because of her hydrophobia; another could not light a stove or sit at a campfire because of pyrophobia. (In the latter case, intriguingly, the fear was accompanied by a fascination with fire and witch burnings.) The Web site www.phobialist.com lists five hundred different specific phobias!

If they didn't cause so much suffering, we could come to appreciate these strange revulsions as touching evidence of the human imagination, like dreams, spontaneous projections from our inner selves. Like dreams, they represent an unbidden release of feelings, thoughts, and physiological symptoms that are experienced as if they were caused from without. Though generated inside us and expressive of our very selves, they are part of that class of experiences about which we say things like "I can't help it" or "It just came over me."

Most small children have a fear of being stared at, and this can reappear in heightened form in a reaction to the stares of animals. Animals themselves react to being stared at as to a threat; a fixed gaze is often a predatory one. This is probably one of the underpinnings of our social phobias and fears of being observed and judged.

No matter what the phobia, the physiological and psychological responses involved originate in the need to defend against a threat. Thus all phobias are connected, at least through metaphor, with the very real dangers of the world. I can assure the reader that when I am in the grip of the fight-or-flight response, I believe that I am dying and that my sanity is draining away and will not be able to reinstate itself. Because of the way the brain works, the thinking in a phobic mind veers toward the catastrophic. Trivial though the cause may be, the associative powers of the mind find analogies for it in the darkest recesses of memory and in the direst interpretations of the world. The sense of doom experienced by the phobic is, in a sense, real, because it is borrowed from the inescapably tragic and dangerous aspects of life, but its application is eccentric.

It is not that the phobic always sees danger where there is none. Most of the sources of phobias, such as means of travel, are not entirely benign, yet the phobic exaggerates the likelihood of problems or feels incapable of tolerating the risk, however small, of a mishap involving them. In many cases one can cure a person of phobias, but one cannot relieve a person of anxiety, since it is an indispensable part of human nature, or, obviously, of the notion that the world is dangerous, as it is.

Both social phobias and simple phobias, even those seemingly trivial—for example, a fear of pigeons, or of crossing the street, or of storms—can have a far-reaching impact on one's behavior and routine. But for many people, phobias are discrete, conquerable responses like psychological allergies, which can be gradually, or sometimes even swiftly, tamed, if not completely unlearned. For some, the phobias are lifelong but not severely incapacitating. For still others, who begin to avoid any situations in which they will or might encounter the objects of their phobias, the original aversions escalate into a serious or even incapacitating restriction of activities, agoraphobia. Apparently some people are prone to react to their phobias in a more global way than others do. They have hair-trigger reflexes to their own responses and find it difficult to revisit the situations in which they have been uncomfortable.

Naturally it is not easy to delineate the exact borderline between being a simple phobic and an all-out agoraphobic. And agoraphobia itself can be more or less extreme: It can manifest itself as difficulty traveling; difficulties going to a mall or restaurant; resistance to doing new things, going to new places, or venturing beyond a specific known area. At its most severe, it can result in the inability to leave home at all or even to leave one room of a home.

Agoraphobia usually begins with a predisposition to panic. Although some dictionaries still use the earlier, more limited definition of "agoraphobia" as simply "fear of open spaces" (the word means "fear of the marketplace" [*phobos* plus *agora-*, "marketplace"]), the clinical category encompasses a large range of experiences. Essentially agoraphobia is a restriction of activities brought about by a fear of having panic symptoms in situations in which one is far from help or escape is perceived to be difficult. It is possible to have agoraphobia without panic attacks, but generally this means only that one has begun to avoid situations in response to the onset of one or two symptoms rather than to the complete cluster of symptoms that is generally experienced in "full-blown" panic.

It was Søren Kierkegaard who, in *The Concept of Anxiety,* first made the distinction between anxiety that had a specific object and anxiety that was simply an emotional or philosophical state. Freud later discriminated among anxiety that was generalized or "free-floating," phobic anxiety, and the anxiety attacks (what we usually today call panic) associated with agoraphobia. Freud, who dreaded train travel, asserted as early as 1895 the basic premise upon which current cognitive/behavioral treatments of agoraphobia rest: "In the case of agoraphobia . . . we often have *the recollection of an anxiety attack*; and what the patient actually fears is the occurrence of such an attack under the special conditions in which he believes he cannot escape it [Freud's italics]."

Panic itself has been much discussed and written about. That it can be both chemically induced and chemically alleviated points to its having a clear biological component. Panic symptoms can be initiated in the laboratory (by the injection of adrenaline, iso-proterenol, or sodium lactate) and can be brought on in life by stress, by substances (such drugs as cocaine and amphetamines or, in some people, caffeine), or even by exercise. While for most sufferers of panic disorder, panic is associated with unfamiliar, stressful circumstances, it can also, in some individuals, occur at inexplicable moments, in familiar surroundings apparently far from stress, and induced in others by its apparent opposite, relax-ation (relaxation-induced panic syndrome). It can occur in sleep (nocturnal panic). It can even be triggered by conventional fluo-rescent lights, which cause a slight sensation of unreality in many people. (Agoraphobics have been shown in controlled tests to ex-perience a raised heart rate and other symptoms in response to a pulsating fluorescent light, possibly enough to trigger panic reac-tions in places, such as supermarkets, where such lighting is used. Newer steady-light forms of fluorescent lighting do not cause these effects.)

The agoraphobe, almost by instinct, arranges to live his or her life within a particular comfort zone, tending to avoid activities or substances that stimulate paniclike symptoms. He feels at risk, as if at risk of sudden death or madness. He commonly seeks the security afforded by carrying perceived safety mechanisms—a cell phone, medicines, food. He may need to go places with a trusted person with whom he feels safe.

The agoraphobe, fearing his own inexplicable physical re-sponses, wants to be near "help." Being in a new environment is a threat because the distance to "help" is no longer known, and the exact topography of fear-inducing situations and objects has not yet been charted.

The reader (and some of my friends and acquaintances) may wonder if I am truly agoraphobic. After all, I do travel, to a degree. I drink coffee, eat chocolate, have a sex life. I even prefer going places—if I have to go—by myself, without a "trusted person." Yet a closer look reveals the guardrails, barriers, and restrictions that have warped my life. Did I get to important family funerals in the West Indies, Chicago, Arizona? To Denmark, Germany, or England to hear my own compositions? Up the elevator to a twenty-fifth-floor apartment to be introduced to a musical colleague I have admired since childhood? To the Springfield Basketball Hall of Fame with my son? No, to all these and many other experiences. For all the things I have done, there are so many more I have opted out of, frozen in my tracks, prohibited not by external circumstances but by a habitual response as concrete as arthritis or an allergy.

It was not always like this, yet reconstructing my hemming in is not simple. Like most children, I was afraid of the dark, a fear I eventually outgrew. But I also had what I now realize were frequent anxiety attacks, starting at around the age of ten or eleven, a few years after my sister had been sent away permanently to what may well have been a better place for her, a school for retarded children. These bouts of anxiety occurred in closed-in situations, in solitude, and often in social settings where one was expected to be still, quiet, and well behaved. I was frequently anxious in class at school, and I felt at such moments as if class were happening to someone else who happened to be me—and a "me" in a state of torture. On the other hand, although I led a somewhat protected life in elementary school and high school, I avoided nothing. I climbed rope ladders, rode roller coasters, went on hiking trips, took the elevator to the top of the Empire State Building, rode the subway, huddled for hours in the back of cold, crowded trucks on winter school trips to the mountains. By the end of high school the number of situations in which I felt acute anxiety had increased. They included elevators and, to a degree, heights and being in the middle of a section of seats in a theater or the backseats of cars that had no back doors. It didn't occur to me to avoid any of these things. I simply endured these episodes of sickening anxiety, which I interpreted as unaccountable physical reactions.

I mentioned nothing about them to anyone, as they had no meaning that I could discern. However, with hindsight I see that my sister's "exile" must have made me reluctant to draw attention to anything that might signify some abnormality in me. Furthermore, the worry that I *was* "abnormal" lurked unconsciously behind my every move, as it does now. My high school roommates knew that I had frequent nightmares and that I was "afraid of death" and afraid my parents would die, normal enough occurrences and feelings. But they didn't know that I left every chorus rehearsal, even of my favorite music—sometimes *particularly* of my favorite music—exhausted from physical tension and torment. As the reader will see, my family life was both unusually supportive and unusually restrictive. While both creative and intellectual expressions were passionately encouraged, outbursts of pure emotion were simply not the family style. Furthermore, there were family secrets and prohibitions that created disturbing undercurrents felt but not discussed. As someone who had grown up trying to decipher my mysterious sister, I was exquisitely attuned to implicit messages about how I should behave. The result was that I held in my feelings and my problems, and they grew without my even knowing it. I wasn't agoraphobic as a child, but following a particularly large number of setbacks right after I graduated from college, I began to rebel against the situations in which I felt terrible. I began to build my life around the experiences in which I felt calm. Fortunately this reining in stopped well short of true incapacitation. Thankfully, I am not like the Englishman I read about recently who could not even walk to the end of his own road and eventually started a business he could conduct on his front lawn.

In a way agoraphobia constitutes a kind of self-allergy. Although to nonphobics agoraphobia is "all in the mind," the physical responses are numerous and can be as manifestly inconvenient as an attack of diarrhea.

Most people I know have phobias of one kind or another. Surely there is no one who has not experienced at least a phobic twinge, whether leaning over the balcony of a friend's thirtieth-floor apartment or suddenly finding a spider crawl up the back of his neck. If this instinctive recoiling is no more than a kind of reflex, like a gag reflex, it will not become a phobia. But if every time you get on the subway you react as if you were being buried alive, you may think twice about taking the subway. You might even begin to feel that subways are dangerous and that people who aren't afraid of riding subways are almost irritatingly blasé about them. For the phobic, if the first response was a strong one, avoidance of the dreaded stimulus when it is next encountered is as natural as a turtle's retraction into its shell when it is hit by a stick.

Until a phobic has undergone treatment specific to the problem, it is hard for him to focus on the fact that his restrictions are rooted in inappropriately learned responses and not in external reality. The response to the external stimulus is simply too quick and too intense to be easily unmasked as a fake, as a false alarm. Since the activated fear reaction is misapplied, the phobic does sense—somewhere deep down—that the danger is inside him and not external. Yet the irrationality of *that* is scary too.

The small child who thinks that there might be a witch underneath his bed is afraid that he might *see* one there, whether or not it is real. To be scared out of his wits, he doesn't need the witch to be real. Quite the contrary, the appearance of a real witch would relieve him of his fear of self, replacing fretful worry with genuine fear. This fear would be entirely directed outward, spurring him to rescue himself.

As in the incident recounted at the beginning of this chapter, realistic fear and phobia can sometimes overlap. After all, the burglar can lock you in a closet. Freud himself notes that "in some cases the characteristics of realistic anxiety and neurotic anxiety are mingled." But that the two reactions are separable within a single personality is borne out by the common observation that phobics often react well in a real crisis, such as those occasioned by war or other emergencies.

An article on the psychological effects of extreme chronic stress written by a doctor, V. A. Kral, who was held in the internment camp of Theresienstadt during World War II, a place where more than thirty-three thousand people died and from which almost eighty-seven thousand others were eventually deported to death camps, suggests that phobias and other neuroses go into a kind of remission under such conditions. The doctor, who worked in the intern-run hospital at the camp, wrote that following an initial period of shock upon arrival, detainees suffered almost universally from depression, apathy, and a pervasive sense of unreality. But panic was rare. Furthermore, he and other psychiatrists were surprised by their observations of "patients who were known . . . from prewar times as suffering from severe and long-lasting psychoneuroses such as phobias and compulsive-obsessive neuroses. These neuroses either disappeared completely in Theresienstadt or improved to such a degree that the patients would work and did not have to seek medical aid. Moreover, no new psychoneuroses developed in the camp." Of such patients who survived the camp ordeal or were not sent east to the death camps, many, although not all, later relapsed into their former neurotic patterns.

The distinction between fear and phobia could be observed in the behaviors of similar neurotic types during the blackouts that have occurred in New York City in the last thirty years and on the day the World Trade Center fell. It was reported by phobia sufferers that during these and similar events their familiarity with anxiety actually acted as preparation for dealing with the emergency. They could in fact reassure others and even rescue others in these circumstances.

In these instances the fear response was monopolized by real danger. As the cause for the fear was plainly real and external, the spiraling psychological terror that accompanies an illogical phobic response was absent. When the mind sought an explanation for the body's emergency posture, it found one readily in the real world and therefore did not fuel the panic process with misguided fears of incipient madness or physical illness. In these cases fear was the body's finite call to action, a tie, however frightening, to the common world shared with others, not the isolating amorphous billowing of some inner unease.

What raises a "character" issue and confuses observers, as well as the sufferers themselves, is that the phobic often responds phobically to situations that cause anyone some stress, impatience, and anxiety (heavy traffic, a crowded elevator). Those who know him assume that he simply lacks the will to face such things. As overwhelmed as they may be by these seemingly innocuous things, phobics do not necessarily lack courage or will in other spheres. A phobia occupies a different plane of experience from fear and normal stress.

Agoraphobia appears to be more common in women than men, perhaps in part for the reason that historically women have had more reasons to remain at home in the first place. If one has a tendency to agoraphobia, an active routine mitigates against its crippling effects, while staying at home can cause a kind of calcification of the tendency. There is ongoing research into the relationship between hormones and phobias. Some phobic women report a reprieve from phobias during pregnancy. But this gender differentiation may well be changing as gender roles in society change. In addition, this data could turn out to be inaccurate. It is well known that men are more reluctant to admit to phobias of any kind than are women.

The first agoraphobics to be studied were in fact men. I learned from Maryanne Garbowsky's impressive study of Emily Dickinson (*The House Without the Door*) that agoraphobia was first mentioned in print in the nineteenth century. From this period date several accounts of male patients who feared walking through empty streets or in open spaces or required companionship to do so or would only venture outside armed with umbrellas or canes. Writing in 1870, Dr. Monitz Benedikt referred to the malady as *Platzschwindel* ("place dizziness"), while a Dr. C. Westphal, writing in 1872, first called it the fear of the marketplace (*die Agoraphobie*). Garbowsky also lists as early names for the illness, *peur des espaces* ("fear of space"), *horreu du vide* ("fear of emptiness"), and "street fear." More recently it has also been called locomotor anxiety and panphobic syndrome.

An 1871 article by Cordes described the symptoms of anxiety occurring in such patients as including palpitations, nausea, headache, chest pain, and shortness of breath. Adding that the anxiety was brought on by being in crowds as well as in open spaces, Cordes pointed out that it was induced by the patient's own thoughts, rather than by the external environment. Indeed the state of mind has sometimes been called endogenous phobic anxiety, meaning that it originates primarily in the person's own nature. Its common accompanying psychic symptom, the disorienting but transient state known as depersonalization, is sometimes called phobic anxiety depersonalization syndrome.

Sometimes the onset of agoraphobia is triggered by a shock or a loss or a death that has made the sufferer vulnerable, and from which, as it were, a general feeling of horror and strangeness is channeled into concrete life circumstances. An agoraphobic named Vincent, writing in 1919, recounted that "after a boy in the village was murdered I almost feared to be alone, was afraid to go into the barn in the daytime, and suffered when put into bed in the dark. . . . There was a high hill not far from my home in the country where we boys used with other boys to coast in the winter time. One evening, while coasting, in company with other boys in the neighborhood, I experienced an uncomfortable feeling each time we returned to the top of the hill. . . . I likewise commenced to dread anything high . . . I even had a fear of crowds of people, and later of wide streets and parks."

Agoraphobia is considered a neurosis and is listed in psychiatric and medical texts as a type of anxiety neurosis. Unlike simple phobias and social phobias, which often begin at an early age, the more global condition of agoraphobia tends to strike people on the cusp of independent adulthood. It bears no connection to psychosis or schizophrenia, although at one time it was erroneously considered a form of schizophrenia. It is not a personality disorder or character disorder. However, it overlaps with other types of anxiety neurosis, such as obsessive-compulsive disorder, in its magical assigning of the feeling of safety to certain places or activities and its triggering of unwanted thoughts. Some phobic behaviors acquire the kind of ritualistic character we associate with a compulsion. For example, a somewhat phobic woman of my acquaintance who had recently moved from the East Coast to the West became incapable of making left turns in her car. To stave off anxiety, she had to contrive to get everywhere by a process of right-hand turns, no matter how convoluted the resulting travel route. One could speculate that an insecurity about the move had expressed itself as a grotesquely exaggerated sensitivity to driving space. By "hugging the shore" of the right-hand sidewalk, she avoided the increased vulnerability to oncoming traffic and wider distances of being in the left-hand lane.

The compulsive relieves his anxiety by performing a particular activity, such as washing his hands repeatedly, after which he feels safe. The agoraphobe can feel safe only under certain conditions or in certain locations and avoids those circumstances that cause anxiety. Presumably this tendency is to some degree universal. Most people feel initially uncomfortable or self-conscious in a new school, a new job, an unfamiliar country, and even, to a minor degree, being in any new surroundings. Along with some fear, most people react to these experiences with what they call excitement. Fear and excitement share many of the same physiological symptoms. But for the agoraphobe the reaction to the unfamiliar can be extraordinarily exaggerated and fundamentally negative.

Phobias and superstitions can overlap. Both represent a misuse of our ability to determine causality between events. In a phobia we mistakenly determine that the cause of our distress is an external experience when the problem is internal. In a superstition we have deduced from anecdote or personal incidents that a black cat crossing our path causes bad things to happen. Once we are confirmed in such associations, disentangling truth from fiction can be difficult. Such beliefs can even influence events. The composer Arnold Schoenberg, who was superstitious about the number thirteen (triskaidekaphobia), regularly made mistakes in his musical scores when he came to the thirteenth page or thirteenth measure.

Everyone I have ever met has difficulties of one kind or another and even phobias of one kind or another, yet it is still difficult to admit to having this condition, in part because it is so difficult to describe. It is even difficult to remember that one has it. At my desk or at the dinner table, in front of my piano, or in a classroom, I don't feel agoraphobic. This may be the result of my being lucky enough not to have what psychiatrists call trait anxiety—or generalized anxiety. I'm anxious only in specific situations (state anxiety). I tend to think of my problem as consisting of specific phobias, whereas actually the condition is a complex network of phobias that constitutes a major handicap.

The person with agoraphobia knows that most of the dangers he avoids are "imaginary" and is ashamed not only of his phobias but of what would appear to be his cowardly and furtive attempts to avoid them. He worries that he will be thought crazy.

Agoraphobia is isolating. Dealing with a mysterious inner threat, the agoraphobe begins to monitor himself most of the time, like the child who fears his own imagination in the dark. Agoraphobics can easily become overly self-absorbed. They can become willing to sacrifice almost anything rather than face the prospect of panic. However, there are also moments when real life forces a choice between inner and outer threat, and outer threat overrides the phobia: when a child is hurt, a parent is dying, an injustice demands that you speak out or show up somewhere dreadful. In general, the agoraphobe suffers from terrible guilt about all the occasions and opportunities lost or marred by his responses and by the unexplained absences or departures that have hurt his relationships. For obvious reasons, then, agoraphobia can be associated with additional problems, such as depression and alcoholism. It can overlap with hypochondria. Although the physical manifestations of the phobic response are not in and of themselves damaging, in the long term severe stress is. Indirectly, then, the pressures associated with being severely phobic can injure one's health. Therefore, even if he is not cured, a sufferer can potentially improve his health by better understanding, and therefore better withstanding, the disorder itself.

The more you examine a subject, the more complicated it seems. When, in passing, you notice a fly on the table, it seems to be only "a bug." If you decide to study it more closely, you enter the vast universe of entomology. The insect, however, stays exactly the same. Only the intensity of your attention has changed.

I now know just enough about phobias to see that they are immensely complicated. They involve both physical and mental symptoms, and these cannot be entirely separated from each other. They are two aspects of our experience that form a continuous loop, and both are registered in the same organ, the brain. It is this loop that has to be dealt with when psychological problems are discussed. Even Freud never thought that psychology began and ended in exclusively mental activity. While our genes predetermine some aspects of our destiny, our bodies and minds are also molded and formed by what occurs to us and are changed by our histories, including the histories of our thoughts and feelings. It is now known that what you feel, experience, and do changes your brain. What you learn becomes a part of you, making the history of your quirks and habits that much more difficult to uncover.

The process of coping with phobias or unlearning them therefore appears to be better understood than how they are acquired or to what degree they are acquired and to what degree they are innate. To what extent do we learn to be phobic or are we born phobic? Which comes first, physical anxiety, life experiences, an innate mental predisposition? How do genetics and evolution figure into the story? When we flee a benign object in terror, are we fleeing the object, its symbolic meaning, or the sensation of terror itself? Are phobias simply a flaw in nature—like flat feet or lower back pain—or do they have a good side? These are questions I can only raise, not answer. And for each of us the balance of answers may be different.

Chapter Two

Father

I stepped from plank to plank
A slow and cautious way
The stars about my head I felt
About my feet the sea.

I knew not but the next
Would be my final inch—
This gave me that precarious gait
Some call experience.
—EMILY DICKINSON

Emily Dickinson's entire body of work seems to issue from a world in which cycles of panic are a constant: the threat of it, the engulfing experience of it, the recovery from it, finally its recollection and the anticipation of its return. Part of the poignancy of her plight is that she did not have any medical context in which to place her extreme dread. For the second half of her life, from the age of twenty-five until her death at the age of fifty-six, she remained essentially a recluse in her home in Amherst, Massachusetts, leaving the area only twice for trips to Boston to see an eye doctor. An agoraphobic, at least in behavior, she suffered from a fear that was mystical and ultimate, with the threat of what felt like true insanity ever present. At the same time, had she viewed her problem from a less personal angle, her poetry would have, at the very least, been transformed. Perhaps it would not have existed.

> I lived on Dread—[she wrote]
> To Those who know
> The Stimulus there is
> In Danger—Other impetus
> Is numb—and Vitalless— . . .

The whole question of psychological diagnosis is fraught with difficulties and is to a degree a matter of interpretation. So-called neuroses form part of a continuum involving anxiety, depression, and compulsions. Agoraphobia is not German measles. In Emily Dickinson's case, for example, John Cody writes that a number of diagnoses might be appropriate depending upon what one considers "the core of her trouble." Among these are "the Adjustment Disorders, Avoidant Personality Disorder, Brief Reactive Psychosis, Cyclothymic Disorder, Depersonalization Disorder, Dysthymic Disorder, Generalized Anxiety Disorder, Hysterical Personality Disorder, Major Depressive Episode, Schizoaffective Disorder, Schizotypal Personality Disorder, and Social Phobia." Furthermore, the understanding of the genetic underpinnings of conditions once deemed to be simply habits is continually evolving. It is now theorized by some, for example, that the irresistible compulsion to continually pull out one's own hair—tricholomania—an affliction that can leave sufferers almost bald, may result from a flaw in the gene connected to grooming.

I suppose that in both my father's and my case phobias might someday be diagnosed as an incidental outcome of some underlying mental abnormality that has yet to be defined. In my childhood I knew that my father suffered from phobias and anx-iety. But in those days no one would have said that his phobias added up to a more general mind-set or that they constituted a "disorder." Like Dickinson, my father did not really have a way to describe his problem. Growing up when American psychol-ogy was still primarily Freudian and visits to a psychiatrist were generally secret, he lived in a milieu of people who were either staunch adherents of Freudian theory or mocking opponents of it. He himself was psychologically inclined, but I am not sure how literally he took Freud's concepts or whether he applied ideas like the inferiority complex and the Oedipus complex to himself. I also tend to think that he kept at arm's length any awareness that his anxiety connected him with the animal king-dom, just as he did the exact way food got to his dinner table.

Today I would say that like me, he was agoraphobic and suf-fered from panic disorder. Unlike Dickinson, he was active and needed the excitement of being out in the world, but he also sought safety and tried to make a safe haven of each context he entered. He saw the magazine he edited as a kind of intellectual and moral haven for its readers. He described each issue as a kind of "present" sent to the subscribers, a reward, perhaps, for making it through the week.

He also needed a high degree of predictability—order. He was a highly compartmentalized man whose natural bent was to live in a structured and restricted way. He was a creature of routine. It made sense that he would put out a magazine every seven days for thirty-five years. He traveled to Europe once, on his honey-moon in 1929. But after a brief return to his home in Chicago, he spent the remainder of his life in Manhattan and Westchester, with the exception of a few forays into known destinations in New England and upstate New York and a handful of trips by train to Chicago to see his relatives. He knew how to drive but made any lengthy trips with others at the wheel, driving his car himself only in the summer and, even then, never farther than the mile or so it took to get from the house he rented in July and August in Bronxville, a suburb only half an hour from New York City, to the stationery store to buy the evening paper or to the movies. On one of these outings with my mother and brother and me in the car, he couldn't get our 1950 Dodge to climb a particularly steep hill. He bravely suggested that the three of us get out and seek help, and we ended up flagging down a policeman, who dramatically backed the car down the incline, with my father, looking stricken, sitting next to him in the passenger front seat. No doubt this experience confirmed him in his ways.

After early middle age he never drove through long tunnels, across sizable bridges, or through new neighborhoods. He avoided most elevators and most upper-floor locations and was able to convince his employers to retain a manually operated elevator at the magazine so that he didn't have to ride in the automated ones. When he took taxis, he instructed the drivers on the route he expected them to take. He did not ride the subway, and he did not ride on buses. He never once traveled by airplane.

Off limits were discussions of blood, disease, and death. If he got a paper cut on his finger, he paled at the sight of the blood and headed nervously to the bathroom for a Band-Aid. His distress at the mention of blood seemed to extend outward to a whole range of topics related to the physical. As children we gradually became accustomed to medical problems being mentioned either euphemistically (". . . something women go through") or with a squirming lack of specificity (". . . after being very sick"; ". . . some sort of terrible illness . . ."). In retrospect, it would appear that he had a severe case of blood injection phobia, which caused the symptoms he suffered when medical subjects arose in conversation, but at the time I thought of this almost as a form of politeness and discretion on his part. On more than one occasion at parties at home he reacted to a medical reference by getting flushed, leaving the room, and retiring to the bedroom to lie down. This apparently happened to him at other people's houses and at work too. Once, when as a young adult I had seriously cut my finger with a kitchen knife and had thirteen stitches in it, I had to remember to mention it to him jauntily as "just a minor thing."

His squeamishness seemed at times to extend to the body itself, although it certainly didn't impinge on his admiration for beautiful women. The subject of how bodies actually work, or fail to work, was discussed euphemistically, as if we were discussing some distant matter accessible only to specially trained experts, not as if this "distant" subject were our very selves. He was not therefore someone who talked much about his ailments or aches and pains. Neither of my parents was a complainer—surely a good thing. But conversely, there was no way for them to come to terms with their physical selves or to "model" this coming to terms for their children. Although affectionate, my father tended to be visibly wary of physical contact and seemed to wash his hands more often after an encounter with a potentially dirty object or hand than would be customary. He looked vaguely appalled when someone coughed in his vicinity, although his natural courtesy made him suppress the look. He tended to pick up small objects with only his pinkie and fourth finger and in conversation would tilt away from rather than toward the person he was speaking to, even if he was in conversation with an alluring woman. He wasn't someone who would taste something from someone else's plate, and he certainly wouldn't share your glass or fork, if so offered. While not precisely a hypochondriac, he responded with extreme caution to the symptoms he felt, while avoiding hearing clinical details that might only make him picture his own inner machinery with greater clarity.

Although when I looked into my father's face, I felt that he had a powerful awareness of his place in nature, he radiated the sense of needing to be protected from the elements. He was highly susceptible to cold and could wear wool sweaters and an overcoat even in summer. He abhorred drafts. Air conditioners caused him muscle stiffness, and he preferred any degree of sweltering New York heat to an air-conditioned space. He seemed fragile when he was in the country and away from his beloved Manhattan. He looked surprised and vulnerable standing on grass and not on pavement. I believe that he found even the sight of mountains and forests somewhat disturbing.

Throughout his life he also suffered from "vertigo," a term in little use these days, a symptom hard to disentangle from those associated with anxiety. It more than likely related to a purely physical condition such as an inner-ear abnormality. If so, neither my brother nor I inherited it. A mild heart attack, suffered when he was in his mid-sixties, shook him deeply, and the fear of a recurrence interlaced itself insidiously with his tendencies to avoid experiences that would cause him anxiety.

He had a temper, all the more threatening because so rarely displayed. He lacked the ability to casually blow off steam. You might say that getting angry or upset frightened him, so that he held his anger inside to an unhealthy degree. In his case the kinds of caustic remarks, bursts of annoyance, or building impatience that might, in some people be a frequent, and also limited, expression of irritation already forecast a full-fledged attack of rage. Even these first tremors were so surprising that in their presence one felt like fleeing for the hills.

He had what might in retrospect seem like a strong streak of social phobia. In addition to avoiding crowded places and always sitting on the aisle and near an exit in any theater or concert hall, he avoided most parties and get-togethers. I don't remember his ever instigating a party on his own. Rather he seemed a somewhat reluctant, passive participant in a social gathering though he usually ended up being the quiet epicenter of the event. He would walk into even his own living room rather tentatively if it contained guests, looking cheerful and ruddy-faced but also hanging back. Though he spent all day with people, they seemed to astonish him. His respect for the complexity and mystery of others was part of what made him a deep person, but it also expressed some inner fear.

Both fascinated and repelled by the physical, he did not carry himself proudly, like someone identifying himself with his body—a sheriff, say, walking into a saloon—but rather hesitantly, with a slightly simian stoop, like someone who was at ease with his mind and with what he had to say but was slightly ashamed or even mystified that he had been born into physical, animal form. When in an expansive mood, however, he stood straight, with his hands characteristically akimbo, conveying a strong magnetism, and when possessed by a sudden thought or in a hurry, he could walk with powerful energy and determination. He was, in a word, physically paradoxical, radiating at one and the same time meekness and a suppressed passion and energy.

He was famously shy, preferring to speak to individuals rather than to a group. But he wasn't shy about expressing deep feelings and convictions or about spending much of his day in conversation with a series of potentially very intimidating individuals. He was in fact surrounded by people at almost all times, and clearly needed to be. I believe that his loneliness was so all-pervasive that the company of others never entirely distracted him from it. He never once that I know of took a solitary trip or even solitary walk, in order "to be alone"; perhaps he already was alone enough. He had, I believe, no actual fear of anyone and in a sense was profoundly sociable. He just needed certain conditions in which to reveal his sociability, just as he needed certain conditions in which to assert himself, to be spontaneous, and to reveal his pride in himself.

His voice was rather high-pitched, with an almost feathery tunefulness, though also unmistakably male. He tended to speak with a measured calmness. His inner nervousness was coupled to a dislike of agitation. His life consisted of a series of intimate tête-à-têtes, his attention centered squarely on the person with whom he was speaking. His care with syntax and word choice was so consistent that I am sure even in a dire emergency he would have shouted for help in excellent English. Once when we were staying at a hotel in Boston, my brother and I were awakened by our father saying, "Boys, there's a fire next door, and we will all need to take the stairs down to the street," which he said as if he were saying that it was time for breakfast. The flames were in fact clearly visible from our window, and inasmuch as he had a morbid fear of being trapped in a fire, he must have been terrified. At the same time, perhaps since this was the real thing, his terror didn't waste time spinning its wheels but evaluated the danger swiftly and rationally.

Despite everything going on inside him, he was a comforting paternal figure to many people. He was a strong, charismatic man, who had great leadership abilities. He seemed to lead through a combination of brilliance, vision, moral authority, kindness, vulnerability, and gentleness. He saw life as essentially tragic and tended to treat people the way the character Alyosha in Dostoevsky's The Brothers Karamazov recommends: "like patients in a hospital." His own extreme sensitivity made him extraordinarily empathic. He cried more easily than any adult I have known, and his crying was audibly expressive of a kind of bottomless sympathy and grief. Tears could be brought on by a life event or something he watched in the theater or TV. The last thing I usually saw as the train pulled out of Grand Central, carrying me to high school in Vermont or later on to college, was the face of my father waving and crying.

Obviously, his shyness and indirectness were expressed most clearly in the role of editor. In this work, his artistry and conviction and will could have an important outlet, but at an angle, without his own name needing to be signed beneath the result. He had, one might say, mixed feelings about having a "self" at all, just as he had mixed feelings about having a "body." It was perhaps not a coincidence that he worked at a magazine that published its articles without a table of contents for so many years, had its articles signed below the last line rather than after the title, and used, in "The Talk of the Town" section and in its obituaries, the collective "we" in place of an undersigned "I." He wrote a great number of those unsigned pieces himself (particularly obituaries) over the years.

At work not everyone was charmed by the obliqueness of his style, in which authority was all the more difficult to challenge because it was so subtly and almost passively employed. This apparent passivity was expressed in the way he described events that he had himself brought about or judgments he had made: "I'm afraid that it just didn't work out" or "For many reasons it was decided . . ." This could be maddening. It also related to his phobias in the sense that a phobic could be said to be viewing his own projections as external forces.

He had a powerful central core and confidence about his judgment, as well as wide intellectual and artistic horizons, which he didn't hesitate to expand continually. In his own way he could be experimental and adventurous and even wild, but admittedly only under special conditions, within the confines of the life he had constructed. Intellectually he was the contrary of agoraphobic. He loved hearing about wildness and adventurousness and took enormous pleasure in seeing people cut loose in movies or on television or in the arts. He loved music, particularly jazz, and could improvise passionately at the piano. However, his sense of improvisation in life was minimal. The structure and routine of that life remained remarkably unchanged for his last forty years. He was at the opposite extreme from someone who would, for example, like the travel writer Edward Hoagland, buy a one-way ticket to a remote African township and arrive without reservations or very much money, just to see what he would discover there.

As is publicly known, from the time he was about forty-three (and I was about two) until his death at eighty-five, he had a second love relationship outside his marriage, which gave his daily routine some of the characteristics of a double life. It was only double viewed from the outside, of course. To him it was just his life. His additional partner, a writer at the magazine, had an adopted son, and it wasn't uncommon for him to eat, or at least, *attend* four or even five meals a day to accommodate all the important people in his life. Few could have sustained the compartmentalization this life required, and it reveals much about his character. That the situation had a profound effect on the development of my phobias I do not doubt, but because it remained a secret from me throughout my childhood, the impact was indirect. My mother never got over the change and couldn't bear the thought that her children would hear of the relationship. My father and I didn't discuss it until his last years. But through it all my parents' marriage did not either end or wither. There must have been terrible tensions, but there did not seem to be a lack of mutual love. It would appear that the primal cell of my father's impulse to domesticity had replicated and that the first cell had survived too. Incredibly, I didn't learn about this dual existence until I was almost thirty. But the secrecy itself and the atmosphere it created are surely relevant to the evolution of my phobias.

In terms of my father's own phobias the implications of this expanded routine would appear to be manifold. For one thing, it supports my suspicion that he dreaded being alone. Clearly, he rarely was. And this relationship helped make the magazine a kind of second home. In fact he kept *both* women fully informed about his whereabouts at all times. So in a sense, as a vulnerable person, he was being doubly monitored as well as doubly loved. In addition, one could say that the situation revealed that his large and passionate nature, which feared itself, needed control, and dreaded conflict, also sought expansion and indeed found a way to expand—an outlet for additional sides of his personality—that was within reach. The additional home added, as it were, an extra loop to the closed circle in which he lived. The period in which the relationship started was one in which enormous burdens descended, among them the new demands of being fully in charge of a major magazine and the sad challenge of having a daughter who was mentally retarded. If this branching out from his original family gave him some relief or escape from these burdens, it also may have helped him to shoulder them. In addition, he extended his own reach further into the world by finding yet another partner who could venture where he did not.

The consequence in my childhood home was to add another thick layer of "discretion" and denial to the many layers that already existed. As the incubating environment for a future adult with travel phobias, the friendly, warm, invitingly scruffy, and (appropriately) rose-colored living room could hardly have

been more ringed by intellectual fence posts. Part of its very appeal to family friends was an atmosphere of delightful predictability. Things seemed very informal, yet at the same time,
the wonderfully high spirits that prevailed when guests appeared
were expressed along circumscribed lines. And the guests tended
not to vary. Although there could be the occasional angry out-
burst on the part of visitors—usually aided by scotch, vermouth,
or a martini—there were few mentions of the magazine, none
of money, very few of being Jewish, almost none of my sister,
and, of course, understandably, none of my father's complex
personal life. The silence on this last topic was airtight, and guests
who might have blurted out something about it—those who
were unpredictable, confrontational, or perhaps too worldly—
were infrequent visitors. Thus it was not only medical subjects
that were avoided. Politics was probably the dominant topic, and
music, led by my father at the piano, became a kind of balm that
seemed to release a good feeling among everyone and give him a
way to express himself that was unguarded, candid, intimate, and
even boisterous. Since my parents did not smoke, and, apart from
an occasional celebratory sip of champagne or, for my father a
medicinal dose of Dubonet, did not drink, their offer of alcohol
and cigarettes to guests conveyed, somehow, an atmosphere of
almost illegal licentiousness, as if our home had suddenly been
transformed into a speakeasy. But the wildness was contained.

Parties may not have been my father's idea, but they are central memories of my childhood. As a five- or six-year-old, lying
in my bed a hallway away from this smoky, tinkling hubbub, I
remember most of all the sound of my mother's high-pitched
laugh as it sailed above the tumult of sophisticated lower voices,
like a soprano above a chattering throng in a Verdi crowd scene.

My father's sensitive nature sometimes protected him. Although I have read and been told of people getting angry *at*

him, I never once witnessed such a thing. Nor did I ever blow up at him myself. The most I ever did was to defy his wishes, and that happened only a few times. I felt extremely comfortable with him, but perhaps even more than is common between parent and child, I adjusted my way of speaking and quite a bit of the content of what I said when I was with him.

All families have their routines, rules, secrets, and taboos. What may have been truly unusual in our family was the degree to which the lid was kept on so much passion and drama, while also appearing *not* to be on. We were in a kind of cheerful pressure cooker. As a small child I was fully aware of the tragedy of my sister—it was staring me in the face—but unable to talk about it. I was only dimly aware of my father's difficulties with anxiety and completely incognizant of my mother's troubles. Subconsciously I must have registered the marital drama, but consciously I would never have tried to root out the causes of any awkwardness I detected in the family routine; such moments simply pointed to puzzling aspects of my parents' personalities. If phobias involve a disturbance in one's reading of reality—the imagining of danger where there is none—in my childhood I learned to *distrust* my nervousness about disturbances beneath the surface of my childhood, where there *were* in fact some deep disturbances. I picked up seismic messages of danger, but there was no outward confirmation that we lived on a fault line. There was a feeling of claustrophobia, of being encased in something, but when I looked up, the blue sky appeared to be right overhead.

Cheerfulness that masks hidden anguish can be even more frightening than the messy truth. From my perspective now, the idea that as a child I felt the presence of dragons at the end of each corner of the known conversational world seems relevant to the development of my agoraphobia. That so much was off-limits seems pertinent to my current dread of exploring the unknown. But it also seems nonsensical for me to blame this or any other aspect of my childhood for my phobias. There are too many close relatives with similar problems. My father, uncle, aunt, and paternal grandmother didn't have my childhood, but they suffered from some of the same fears I do. I may make connections between the stresses and traumas of childhood and what I experience now, but these seem merely one part of a complex weave of thought, emotion, behavior, and physiology, rather than the source of the condition.

My father's phobias may have deeply disturbed him at one time, but at least by the time he had children, they seemed to have become simply a part of his interesting character. His restricted radius of activity seemed to have about as much bearing on his sense of self-esteem or his sense of being fully alive as J. S. Bach's limited travel experience had on him. Of course Bach was no phobic, and in fact he once walked fifty miles to hear the famed organist and composer Dietrich Buxtehude perform. But he saw even less of the geographical world than my father did.

As I age, I see more and more how much anguish my father must have endured. I also remember his brave attempts to make it to events involving my brother and me or to stay through them when they were in difficult settings. Once, when my brother and I were already adults and presenting a short opera in Lenox, Massachusetts, on which we had collaborated, he hired a car to drive him there, got only as far as Brewster, New York, and turned back. Such moments surely pained him.

Overall I believe that the tensions and paradoxes of his nature were rather successfully balanced as if in some kind of psychic isometric exercise. Still, I can't help thinking that there was something deeply unresolved in his nature that confronted him when he was isolated, trapped, or far from the familiar. In other words, his phobias were perhaps fueled, at least in part, by all that he had difficulty acknowledging in himself and expressing directly.

The degree of my admiration for my father—the fact that I hoped to be like him in his better aspects—may have been a contributing factor in my annexation of his problems. When you love someone, you can pick up his mannerisms. I once had a similar reaction to a composition teacher of mine who had a stammer. During the period in which I studied with him I would sometimes find myself stammering when I was talking about music with friends. I had acquired his speech difficulty along with his excitement about music

If my father thought about the development of his personality, he didn't have much to say about it at home. But we all knew that his own father, Benjamin, had been an adventurous, enterprising, extroverted man whose entire life was a demonstration of a nonphobic temperament. Ben's parents had emigrated in the late nineteenth century from Warsaw, Poland. Ben ran away from home as a teenager, performed roles as an actor in a traveling troupe, and started his own business, selling jackknives and jewelry at the age of sixteen. He began with a cart of wares which he transported by horse and buggy through remote regions of Ontario and the American West, and ultimately built a prosperous firm housed in Chicago's famed stockyards, the origin, perhaps, of his youngest son's lifelong aversion to blood. He liked traveling (I remember seeing photos of him kissing the Blarney stone in Ireland) and was spontaneous, explosive, sometimes bawdy, and direct.

By contrast, my father's mother was quiet, cultivated, and, it is rumored, somewhat phobic. It would appear that psychologically my father grafted many aspects of his father's domineering and venturesome personality onto his mother's introspective, poetic, and more cautious disposition. Presumably any chemical or genetic predisposition to phobia was passed to my father from the maternal side.

At least two of my father's siblings, his brother Mike, to whom he was very close, and his sister Melba, suffered from phobias. In fact my father saw terribly little of Mike in their last years because of their common fear of flying. Mike lived in Chicago. Like many phobic people, he had a nonphobic partner, who, wonderfully, helped him brave the trip to my parents' fiftieth wedding anniversary in 1979.

As the baby of the family, the youngest of five children, my father had been coddled and overprotected. The family's affluence further shielded him and fostered his reliance on others. For a time his parents had a chauffeur, who helped initiate his lifelong automotive dependency. The few times I saw my father with his relatives later in life I always thought that however pleased and relaxed he was with them, he felt obliged in their presence to hold in check his strongest attribute, his intellect. Living in a rowdier and less rarefied world than he did, they regarded his mind with awe. But he seemed almost embarrassed to reveal to them how much he had grown and made himself look slightly reduced as a result, once again the youngest and most delicate of the group of siblings. Nonetheless, he always seemed to enjoy this shedding of his current skin.

My father became bookish at an early age, a young man of words, of thought, feeling, and language—but not of action. He never learned to cook himself a meal and certainly not to change a tire. He regarded with suspicion most machines, even simple ones like toasters.

His general apprehensiveness also began early. His father's temper apparently frightened him, as did the gore and animal suffering on view in the stockyards and perhaps, one could speculate, the very implements his father sold. While still in elementary school, he was shocked when the brother of one of his best friends, a neighbor from down the street, was murdered in a calculated plot by older boys, one of whom attended the same school as my father. It was even rumored that the teenaged murderers, who became legendary as Leopold and Loeb, might have considered making my father's brother Mike their victim. Therefore my father was—at least in imagination—only one or two steps away from being the victim himself. Equally important, he was only a few steps away from the violence and warped sensibilities of the perpetrators.

The sense that something terrible was about to happen always hovered over my father. One of his few signed pieces as a young writer concerned the imagined devastation of New York City by a meteor, and he determined that John Hershey's *Hiroshima* should occupy an issue of the magazine empty of all other articles and of cartoons; and he spent several decades contemplating the effects of nuclear war on the planet. On the one hand, the global reach of my father's dread was the height of rationality and clearsightedness. Nothing could be more foolhardy than to look away from the horrors of the world and to see no danger where there is so much. But more than many people, and more than might have pleased him, he also seemed to carry the world's dangers within him, and his sensitivity to them combined with a dread of some of life's more potentially positive experiences.

The paradox is that without his phobias he would not have achieved what he did. He might well have achieved other things, which might possibly have been more gratifying to him, but not what he proved so masterful at. In his twenties he had written a number of popular songs and music for modern dance productions. Since he wrote and played only by ear, my mother was his music copyist in these musical ventures. During the Depression he composed the score for a musical, *Cabbages and Kings*, which was produced in a small New York theater. His own father turned up unexpectedly there one night—all the way from Chicago—and surprised him backstage with a great bear hug at the end of the show, whereupon they both burst into tears. But as a young composer he was shocked by the cutthroat music world, so far from the artistic climate he had imagined as a young fan of Duke Ellington and George Gershwin. There is even a story in the family that a fellow composer stole the rights to one of his songs. He struggled in a different way as a young writer, fighting to carry out his assignments as a reporter at the magazine despite his shyness and his phobias. Having to travel to New Jersey through the tunnel under the Hudson River or taking a narrow, rickety elevator to cover a story on an upper floor of a tenement must have taken a great deal out of him. (In his book *About Town*, Ben Yagoda called attention to the extraordinarily vivid description of an elevator in one of my father's sets of notes for a reporting piece.) Getting his first job at the magazine was itself achieved anonymously; it was my mother who applied for the position as a reporter for the two of them. Unpublished novels and countless stories by my father remained in his closets after his death. They are exquisitely written. But within them he remains constrained—or so it seems to me—as if impeded at the source by his own reticence.

He blushed easily—blushing is apparently a genetically determined tendency—so he often couldn't help telegraphing the very sensitivities and embarrassments he might have hoped to conceal. He also visibly flinched at being photographed. He seemed to fight off being revealed, known, pinned down.

As an editor he felt free to be himself. Although he felt

creatively frustrated and sometimes imagined leading a different life entirely, it was as an editor that he was fully deployed as a personality, intellect, and creative force and that he was dynamic and decisive. Editing involves to a degree censorship, and he was already a master of self-censorship. But more important, editing is a process of fostering and liberating, freeing both the writer and the writing from whatever holds it back, cutting and pruning and guiding in the service of more exuberant growth. He could free the writing, he could encourage it, he could even help it to run wild—but it wouldn't be his. I remember the amazing energy he exuded when I visited him at the magazine, his apple-cheeked complexion, his surprising sociability. There he did not need to go to people. The world's most fascinating people came to him, bringing news of places he would never dream of going to and of things that enthralled him but would be very difficult for him to investigate firsthand. His immense curiosity mediated between the writer's interest and the reader's need for clarity and literary art. In his editor's chair, his passion for life and his interest in people could be fully expressed. Had he been an inveterate traveler, a doer, or a true extrovert, he would have become too jaded and worldly to maintain the striking innocence and almost infinite receptivity that made him capable of listening so raptly and carefully to what writers had to say. Through his work at the magazine he was able to filter the unruly and terrifying world through his own personality without venturing very far. But while he was able to keep at bay and manage the unknown to some degree, he also carried it within him. This buried volcano of passions and fears created a surface tension that was palpable.

A teacher of mine, the extraordinary composer Earl Kim, once told our class of young composers: "Just remember: Your strengths *are* your weaknesses." I could apply this maxim to my father. His phobias and his accomplishments were inseparable.

Chapter Three

Links in a Chain

Some instances noted at this time [before the earthquake] were of snakes being found frozen on the road, chickens refusing to enter their coops, pigs rooting at their fences, cows breaking their halters and escaping . . . rats appeared to behave as though drunk.
—HAICHENG EARTHQUAKE STUDY (1979) IN *VAN NOSTRAND'S SCIENTIFIC ENCYCLOPEDIA*

Nothing could have been further away from the natural world than my childhood. The windows of our apartment faced Central Park—Olmsted's beautifully tamed and molded version of fields and woods—and trips to the "country" meant journeys to Westchester. At home the nonhuman animal kingdom was represented by the occasional turtle, a pair of goldfish, and briefly a canary. For a year, at the age of about seven, I had a hamster, Sawdust, and his death left me almost speechless with grief, so stunned and embarrassed by the depths of my feelings that I couldn't articulate them.

No doubt in part because of my father's gruesome memories of the stockyards, his squeamishness about blood, and his horror of suffering generally, the animal origins of the foods on our table were unmentionable. Food was simply food. There were two kinds of chickens: living ones and those that came in packages. That these two kinds were one and the same was shrouded behind a veil of secrecy, lest we be forced to become vegetarians. Since my parents were not religious, there was no tradition, other than a kind of spiritualized existentialism, in which to place "nature," and there was no comfortable intellectual space in which to place a discussion of our place in nature. My father seemed to carry the inexplicability of the cosmos around with him everywhere, neither kneeling down to it nor, however warily, embracing it. Every once in a while he would make an effort to address the larger questions that so obviously preoccupied him, without falsifying his lack of "belief." I remember his once quietly commenting, as if making the point to my brother and me once and for all, "We don't know why we have been placed on this earth."

The only way to begin to understand the strange forms anxiety and its effects can take in some people or to comprehend why we have any of the varied, bizarre quirks we have is to retrace our behavior patterns to their roots. We need to remember that we are creatures. The point may seem self-evident, but how can one overstate it? In fact how can we even comprehend it? As brilliant and sophisticated as my parents were, they were so urbanized and so connected from dawn to dusk with the manmade that the world of their creatureliness remained disturbing and subterranean. I am not much different. While driving, I feel a kind of latent terror looking at the effects of the buckling earth visible on the sides of the road. I feel that the comfortable world of my childhood living room, with its scruffy sofas and dust-covered stereo system from the late 1950s, represents reality and that the layers of rock revealed in the sheer sides of roadside cliffs are a kind of affront to that reality.

Strangely, it would appear to be part of human nature to live myopically, regarding ourselves, in some indefinable way as somehow "apart" from nature. In actuality we do not exist "apart" from nature, any more than our hand exists apart from the arm to which it is attached. Though we live surrounded by evidence of our own importance and mostly through newspapers and television and the computer, surrounded by news of things happening today or in the recent past, our egocentrism, ethnocentrism, and chronocentrism are mere coping devices. Indeed they are survival mechanisms. Deep down we may know that we are merely tiny particles in a vast interconnected chain of life, but for the sake of our immediate survival, we don't focus on that fact. While we know full well that everyone on earth has a behind, an anus, and genitals, we tend to feel as if our own were terribly special, a bit embarrassing. In order to fulfill our immediate needs we must be attentive to the present, holding at bay our awareness that we carry within us the chemicals cooked in the early earth, and that at every moment our bodies and minds are perpetuating behaviors refined over millions of years. In moments of relaxation, passion, joy, and fear or when we are confronted by death, injury, or emergencies, this larger context is suddenly reopened for an instant, like a never healed wound.

In fact the entire history of the modern human—*Homo sapiens*—goes back only a minuscule amount of time, perhaps as little as 120,000 years. While our intellectual capacities may have evolved significantly beyond that of the modern ape, we still share with it 98 percent of our genome sequence, the part we each inherited from our common ancestor. We have retained most of the traits we possess for the same reason they were perpetuated through the process of natural selection: We need them. When I turned my car around in the woods, or my father grew uncomfortable in a crowd, or the agoraphobic Vincent blanched at walking through a park, we were exhibiting aspects of the same fight-or-flight reaction an ape experiences when cornered by adversaries in a cave or in an open field where there is nowhere to hide. The notable difference being, of course, that it was not apparent in our cases what or where the dangers were. To understand my unpleasant shadow better I had to read up on how psychologists view this seemingly unhelpful application of fear, on the various ways it is thought one can learn to interpret nonthreatening things as dangerous, and to think about how I came to "inherit" this problem from my father. But first I needed to know how nature intended us to respond to danger, and how the brain coordinates this response.

Darwin made a wonderful study of the expressions of emotions in animals and an accompanying study of the expression of emotions in humans. He distinguished between "animals" and "humans" only for convenience sake. By "physical expressions" he meant both spontaneous outward facial and gestural expressions and their accompanying internal physiological expressions. Humans do have some emotional expressions that animals lack. Among these—and they reveal much about what is distinctively ours—are blushing, weeping, and laughter. (Animals are rarely embarrassed.) But Darwin made the key observation that in the emotions shared by humans and animals, the physical expressions are remarkably consistent. He also observed that for the most part these same expressions are prevalent among long-separated human societies. The data he collected provided evidence that humans' behavior, down to the way we use our hands when we are excited, distressed, or revolted and to the way our stomach feels when we are contented, angry, or frightened is constructed from the same building blocks as those furnishing comparable responses in other primates and mammals. Just as our ability to walk upright derived from tiny changes in the hominid line occurring over millions of years, so our human responses and "expressions" evolved out of those in the animal kingdom. In the human brain and body, new elements were added, but little was removed from this shared past.

The word "emotion" derives from the Latin root *movere*, "to move." Darwin tried to demonstrate that universal facial expressions and bodily gestures expressive of "emotion" have their roots in movements, in actions. "An emotion may be very strong," Darwin wrote, "but it will have little tendency to induce movements of any kind, if it has not commonly led to voluntary action for its relief or gratification."

In his study, Darwin related our involuntary physical and facial expressions to the bodily acts of which they may be residual habits. He related an animal or human crying out in pain to the young of either calling for its parents; the universal downward-turned mouth of disgust as a remnant of vomiting or of spitting out what is noxious; the clenched or pounding fist of anger as a vestige of acts of violence; the common gesture of thrusting one's hands forward in denial as a remnant of the physical act of pushing away, of casting off what is unwanted.

In this work he revealed himself to be a poet of observation. In both animals and humans, for example, he noted that when anticipating pleasure, creatures exhibit a kind of strangely "purposeless" animation. He contrasted the "loud laughter, clapping of hands, and jumping for joy" of children expecting pleasure with the quietude of their actual enjoyment. Commenting that this liveliness may in part reflect the pleasure in "the mere exertion of the muscles after long rest or confinement" or the quickened circulation caused by the excitement of joyful thoughts, he also observed that for many animals the acquisition of most of their pleasures is "associated with active movements, as in the hunting or search for food, and in their courtship." He called this the principle of serviceable associative habits. As infants we reject the mother's nipple by moving our heads to the side. As adults we reject an idea by shaking our heads. Likewise, a man in a passion, "if he tells any one in a loud voice to be gone, generally moves his arm as if to push him away, although the offender may not be standing near, and although there may be not the least need to explain by a gesture what is meant . . . and so in innumerable instances."

Furthermore, said Darwin, these expressions tend also to be functional. The mouth, which opens instinctively in "surprise" in humans, does so because in this position it is capable of taking in the deep breath needed for the strong exertion required to escape or respond. In the instant after being surprised, one almost ceases breathing altogether, so as to hear every sound "as distinctly as possible"; the jaw "drops" from the relaxation of muscles occurring as others tense to confront the cause of astonishment. The widened eyes of surprise have the effect of letting in more light and improving vision. Those who live with animals see this expression when they unexpectedly drop a container: instant alertness, ears up, eyes fully open.

In such cases Darwin saw expressions as being involuntary actions of a directly useful kind. In still other cases he traced expressions to what he termed the principle of antithesis, the notion that if one action customarily accompanies an experience, its opposite, even if "of no use," will tend to arise to accompany the contrary experience. This he attributed to an instinctive reversal of the muscle movements habitually associated with the opposing emotion. He gave as an example the pointed ears, closed mouth, and purring of a cat in an affectionate state, contrasted with its lowered ears, openmouthed growling when it is in fight mode.

Finally he noted, a century before the fuller accounting of

the nervous system we have today, the power of the radiation of "nerve force"—the autonomic nervous system—throughout the body and the multitude of physical and experiential consequences this has.

Regardless of how these mechanisms are filtered through the diversity of individuals, they remain startlingly universal.

When it came to fear, Darwin was particularly eloquent. Himself subject to paralyzing panic attacks as well as to debilitating lifelong psychosomatic ailments, he wrote of fear with profound identification:

> With all or almost all animals, even with birds, Terror causes the body to tremble. the skin becomes pale, sweat breaks out, and the hair bristles. The secretions of the alimentary canal and of the kidneys are increased, and they are involuntarily voided, owing to the relaxation of the sphincter muscles, as is known to be the case of man, and as I have seen with cattle, dogs, cats and monkeys. The breathing is hurried. The heart beats quickly, wildly, violently . . . the strength of the muscles soon fails. In a frightened horse I have felt through the saddle the beating of the heart so plainly that I could have counted the beats. The mental faculties are much disturbed.
>
> . . . Cats, when terrified, stand at full height, and arch their backs . . . they hiss, spit or growl. The hair over the whole body, and especially on the tail, becomes erect.

Explaining that expressions build upon one another, Darwin reminded us that human fear often follows upon astonishment and that as in astonishment, fearful eyes open wide (to see better), eyebrows rise (improving the sense of hearing), and the mouth gapes. He observed the impulse in fear to freeze and almost cease breathing or to crouch low, as if to escape detection. He described the palpitating, loudly audible heart, the "hurried" breathing; the paleness and coldness of the skin, combined with excess perspiration (what we call breaking into a cold sweat), a trembling that begins in the lips and soon takes over the entire body, the relaxation of the sphincter muscles. He connected the dryness of the mouth to the trembling, as a result of which the voice "becomes husky or indistinct, or may altogether fail." He noted that in this state we share the erection of the tiny hairs on the skin (and sometimes the hairs on the head) with many other species, considering this response to be a possible residue of physical changes originally calculated to inspire fear in enemies.

In "an agony of terror," Darwin wrote, the pupils dilate, there is "a gasping and convulsive motion of the lips," the arms may be thrown forward "as if to avert some dreadful danger," and often there is a "sudden uncontrollable tendency to headlong flight." As Freud did some years later, Darwin detailed the differences in phases of fear, beginning with dread (anticipatory anxiety) and culminating in the exhausted collapse following a horrifying experience.

Darwin suffered from terrible anxiety before embarking on his *Beagle* voyage in 1831. But this was nothing compared with his agonies upon his return and for the remainder of his long life. His symptoms, which most scholars now believe had no organic cause, included several belonging to his account of fear: palpitations, extreme gastroenteric distress (flatulence, nausea), and trembling. In addition, he had many of the common symptoms of panic (blurred vision, tingling sensations in the extremities [paresthesia], feelings of faintness, and pains in his chest, as well as a sense of impending catastrophe). During the period in which he worked on *On the Origin of Species* he would awaken trembling in terror in the middle of the night. In his notebooks he described the effects of fear as mimicking those of someone fleeing: "The sensation of fear is accompanied by troubled beating of heart, sweat, trembling of muscles, are not these effects of violently running away, and must not running away have been usual effects of fear." Since he lived two generations before Freud, and the more sophisticated understanding of psychosomatic symptoms Freud's work initiated, he spent decades believing that he suffered from a life-threatening illness. So powerful are the physical symptoms caused by emotional stress that not even Darwin, one of the great minds of science, could evaluate whether his illness was organic or psychosomatic in origin.

Chapter Four

Contemplating the Brain

The brain—is wider than the Sky—
For—put them side by side—
The one the other will contain
With ease—and You—beside
—EMILY DICKINSON

The speck that weighs more than the world.—
—FREDERICK SEIDEL, "JANE CANFIELD (1887–1984)"

Darwin taught us that our internal responses are essentially the same ancient survival mechanisms possessed by our primate ancestors and derived from the long chain of mammalian, reptilian, and amphibian life forms that preceded them. Neurologist and author Antonio Damasio calls these responses "emotions" to distinguish them from the feelings—sentiments, associations, memories, thought patterns—we consciously have about them. These reactions and their physical preparations are innate. As he puts it, ". . . for certain classes of clearly dangerous or clearly valuable stimuli in the internal or external environment, evolution has assembled a matching answer in the form of emotion." Although classes of "dangerous or clearly valuable stimuli" may have changed in the past five millon years, we still need to be on the lookout for anything that could threaten life and limb and to have a keen nose for the things that sustain us. It is a matter of life and death. We respond to such stimuli globally, as entire creatures, in both "body" and "mind."

Our organically embedded responses are activated by the brain. And the way they are activated, which brain areas are involved and the degree to which they are involved—is different for each quality of "emotion." Nowadays one can actually view the neural patterns they make through functional MR imaging, the scanning of the brain in action. (As a musician trying to understand this I have come to imagine each of the primal emotions as differently "orchestrated" in the brain.) Systematic responses as fundamental as the fear response originate in a rather small number of deeply submerged locations in the brain, among them the brain stem region, hypothalamus, and basal forebrain, areas of the brain that predate the vast cognitive networks unique to human beings found in the cortex. From commands originating in these few areas in the brain, the entire body and eventually the feeling and thinking brain are changed in accord with a given emotional pattern. These complex programmed responses lie beneath our behaviors and become overlaid with our personal idiosyncrasies, memories, and thoughts. In creatures with little or no conscious thought, such responses are virtually automatic. They generate instinctive behaviors that preserve and perpetuate their species. Thus, when a baby bird senses a large object flying over its nest, its body activates chemical, neural, autonomic, and motor responses that cause it to make itself as compact and quiet as possible. It does this without, as far as can be determined, any conscious knowledge that it is avoiding the attention of a possible predator. In the same way, many insects instinctively construct nests for descendants they will never encounter.

For humans these global responses take on intricate personal colorations. We are poetic, thoughtful, associative beings. Only factors pertaining to you alone will determine whom you might find sexually attractive. But when you respond this way, the parasympathetic arousal you will experience will have at its core a systemic response, one refined over millennia of slow evolutionary growth, which you share with humans generally. This is the network of reactions that creates the sense of inner tranquillity and the urge to bond sexually and to collaborate with another human being that we call love. This drive to "approach" is almost as hard to resist as is panic's urge to flee. Since it is the very appetite that sets procreation in motion, it is no wonder that when our impulse to get closer to a romantic object is thwarted, we feel wretched. This misery has its analogy in the distress we feel when, in the grip of fight-or-flight symptoms, we are prevented from fleeing. Although each person's thoughts, associations, and behaviors in love are individual, the bodily states involved are universal. For example, a sensation as subtle as the physical buoyancy, or floating feeling, associated with romance is so taken for granted that it can be evoked without explanation in a thousand love songs (e.g., "I have often walked down this street before/ But the pavement always stayed beneath my feet before"). The feeling arises from the chemistry of pair-bonding, attachment, and trust, in which a hormone called oxytocin plays a crucial role, part of the evolutionary glue, as it were, that keeps couples together to raise offspring.

The protective mechanism of disgust is activated as instantaneously as fear. If we reach for a glass of fresh orange juice and by mistake drink from one that has been sitting on the counter for a week, our spitting reaction is almost immediate, ensuring that not much of the stale juice gets digested. If we so much as see someone else in such a situation, our facial expressions mimic the reaction. I saw this response not long ago at the supermarket at the customer service counter. When a lady at the front of the line opened a putrid package to show that the contents were spoiled and couldn't be consumed, it took but a millisecond for everyone in back of her to move away, hold their noses, audibly gasp, and adopt the universal openmouthed scowl of disgust, complete with outstretched tongues and wide-open eyes.

It is interesting that our facial expressions of moral repugnance are drawn from the same repertoire as the physical form and that we describe moral outrage similarly ("Your behavior disgusted me"). Since disgust is an active ingredient in some phobias, particularly those of snakes, spiders, or rodents, it is interesting to see its vocabulary also appropriated for an aversion to disgusting or untrustworthy people, who can be called slimy or who make one's "flesh crawl."

While we learn early to expect and accept the symptoms we experience when we run a mile, or get angry at a friend, and are likely to have had as children a thorough education from friends, family, teachers, books, and movies on the physical reactions associated with sex, we grow up surprisingly ill trained in the physiology of anxiety. Fewer things that happen within us should command greater respect than this response system or have such wide-ranging ramifications.

Although not conscious of their universality, and although they may be quick to mock the more embarrassing symptoms in others, children soon learn the basic human and animal expressions of emotion that Darwin studied. Every child knows that people feel like emptying their bladder or may have diarrhea symptoms when they are nervous. The response makes for low humor in many a children's film. Yet the knowledge is unconscious enough so that when as adults we hear of these reactions in accounts of truly horrific circumstances—in descriptions of concentration camps, or interrogation cells, or slave ships—we are deeply shaken.

Drawing on the child's awareness of this familiar repertoire of symptoms, cartoons are able to exaggerate comically the reactions of fear, while sticking close to Darwin's account of them. When Goofy is confronted with a huge bulldog, his trembling becomes a veritable riot of uncontrollable body movement, his knees knock in salsa rhythm, his chattering teeth leap out of his mouth and fly around on their own, sweat pours like rain from his forehead, he stammers because he is short of breath, and his voice comes out like a squeak. Children seem almost universally to regard the rehearsal of these symptoms as funny, perhaps precisely because they sense the tension between the self-control they are being urged to develop and the aspects of behavior that are automatic. For the same reason children are drawn to animals and instinctively relate to them. If you want to tell a small child a story with a moral, it is likely to communicate all the more readily if the tale concerns a frog or a pig. Apparently children are instinctively aware that they are members of the animal kingdom, while adults instinctively distance themselves from it.

In literature we take for granted the correlation between physical descriptions and the emotions they indicate: "His teeth clenched"; "He stiffened, his eyes widened, and for a moment he stared in disbelief "; "His voice was barely audible"; "His nostrils flared"; "The blood drained from her face"; "She turned as white as a sheet"; "He stamped his foot with rage"; "He pounded his fist"; "He scowled"; "Her eyebrows lifted in surprise"; "His eyebrows lifted in disdain"; "My knees almost buckled under me"; "My knees grew weak when he spoke"; "He shook with fear"; "I stood stock-still, unable to move, or breathe." Such references confirm the universality of our physical expressions of emotion.

When I was small and was first told that my sister was "brain damaged," I found this evidence of the mind's fragility terrifying. I assumed that most people had brains which were intact, whereas my sister's had somehow come unglued. I wondered whether mine was equally vulnerable. At an early age I tried to read up on the brain, but I lacked the aptitude to understand what I read, and the experience induced a kind of vertigo. My brain seemed to flinch at being asked to make sense of its own description, to flee from it, like Dracula from the sign of the cross. My phobia problem has given me an additional reason to delve into the subject, since for good or ill, it is the brain that coordinates the body/mind's responses to the world. Today I grasp the obvious fact that no brain is without its "flaws"; since each forms only gradually in the fetus, and to a degree remains malleable throughout life.

"There is an awful lot that can go wrong in the brain," my friend Michelle, a student of developmental psychology, told me. "There are more connections in the brain than there are stars in the universe. The sheer fact that they come together as well as they do, and as consistently as they do, is amazing.

"We are born with a primal neural repertoire, which ideally means we are born with the ability to do anything that hasn't been constrained by evolution. So we can't fly because evolutionarily we are not designed to fly. But theoretically we can do whatever people can do. But the truth is that no one is born with a completely intact primary neural repertoire. Sometimes there are extreme deficits, but everybody has weird modulations, everybody has strange posturing—how one stands and moves— everybody has weird responses to some things. There are always things that aren't there."

The brain's appearance is relatively nondescript, resembling something between a cauliflower with deep furrows and an elaborately textured powdered wig. When it is cut in half at various angles, its intricate foldings and overlappings are revealed, as are hidden passageways, such as the four ventricles that secrete the nourishing and protective cerebrospinal fluid, and numerous tiny structures shaped like miniature independent organs. I would love to hold one in my hands, as Oliver Sacks does several times in the BBC series *The Mind Traveller*. In one episode, wearing latex gloves, he lifts the slippery organ reverently and tenderly and slices it into thin segments, which resemble white mushrooms.

But although the brain looks like an object, as if it might have one specific function, nothing could be more deceptive. Even if it resembled a miniaturized New York City, with every window in all of its five boroughs lit and full of activity, it would still not suggest the intricacy of its billions of neurons and "several trillion interneuron connections." And nothing that can be seen or held in the hands could possibly suggest the miraculous music that is made inside the brain, a music inaudible outside and heard only by the brain's possessor. For this very reason René Descartes, writing in the early 1600s, proposed that the brain was material but that somehow the "mind" was not. This distinction between "brain" and "mind"—Cartesian dualism—continues to exert great power, despite the important current investigations by researchers Gerald Edelman and Damasio and others into the nature of consciousness.

Consciousness appears to have been a latecomer to the chain of life, probably originating in reptiles no more than 250 million years ago. Creatures from different stages of evolution experienced their sensory faculties differently, depending upon the size and aptitude of their brains. The faculty of vision as it exists in an amphibian is not the same as the vision of the reptile, which possesses, in Oliver Sacks's words, a much more "flowing mobile consciousness" and demonstrates an "active attention" with the ability to perceive a continuity of events and make inferences from past experiences. By contrast, according to Sacks, the consciousness of amphibians is comparatively mechanistic: "The frog does not have a visual world or visual consciousness as we know it, only a purely automatic ability to recognize an insect-like object if this enters its visual field, and to dart out its tongue in response."

Consciousness is also a frequent latecomer—if sometimes only by a few seconds—to the automatic processes that take place in our bodies. The onset of "emotions" as primal as hunger, anger, fear, happiness, and love *precedes* the activation of those complex networks of thought and feeling that eventually reach our awareness even if this onset is triggered by a passing subconscious thought. What we laypeople think of as the body is far faster than the conscious mind. Associations and memories are so deeply, neurologically, physically encoded in us that they trigger physiological responses before the conscious mind is aware. Only then do conscious interpretations, memories, sentiments, and associations get into the act. As Freud predicted, the brain, and so consciousness, operates on many different levels simultaneously.

Evolution is a history of building and adapting. Like everything organic in nature, the brain developed over aeons of time and, housed in countless species, passed through many stages. The embryo developing in the womb almost seems to recapitulate some of the earlier stages of evolution, as does its developing brain. Like the layered geology of the earth, the adult human brain contains its own history. At the bottom, connecting to the spinal cord, is what biology teachers call the reptilian brain or sometimes the old brain or the brain stem. Much of this pre-conscious ancient portion of the brain is indistinguishable from the brain structures found in a lizard, in which it also regulates motion, sight and smell.

Above this is the mammalian part of the brain, correspon-ding more to the brains found in early mammals. This houses the limbic system, the seat of many of our most elemental emotional responses and intense memories, which includes the thalamus (meaning "marriage bed"), a crucial center for communication and coordination of the information gathered by our senses, as well as the all-important amygdala. The amygdala, in addition to being a storehouse of primitive and intense memories and a cen-ter for response to threats, is crucial for the attachment of emo-tional significance to things. It is largely responsible for the chemistry associated with experiences of passion, rage, crying, and consolation. Almost everything that happens in the brain and in the rest of the body passes through this limbic system, but it also contains its own direct routes to the peripheral nervous system, so that it can generate nearly instantaneous responses to external stimuli before the upper "cortical" sections of the brain begin to process what is happening.

As mammals evolved, the coordination in the brain between the senses became increasingly sophisticated as a new layer, the cor-tex, grew above the old reptilian brain and the limbic system. The cortex underwent its greatest expansion in the primates from which *Homo sapiens* evolved, with the brain reaching about one-third its current human size in *Australopithecus africanus* three mil-lion years ago. A dramatic enlargement of the cortex and then the neocortex occurred in hominids about 1.5 million years ago, caus-ing the raising and flattening of forehead and "domed scull" of our hominid ancestors, bringing with it an exponential increase in "thinking, planning, organizing and communicating." Language in turn almost doubled the size of the frontal lobes in *Homo sapiens*, as brain tissue expanded to store and coordinate all the new information it was receiving and engage in the activities the cortical portions of the brain made possible.

Thus the cortex and neocortex in our brains sit atop two other basic brain structures, the main functions of which antedate human existence. Our brains embody a history of millions of years. Our thought processes, those of which we are aware and even those vast territories that pass beneath the radar of our consciousness, issue from the recent parts of our brain. But beneath them is a vast silent world of impulses, feelings, and coordinated life responses.

This description of an organ that through evolution eventually began to ponder its own existence gives off an eerie familiarity. It is a progression reproduced in the tale of the Garden of Eden. It is almost as if that long transition during which the old reptilian brain, which simply *acted,* grew its new section, the cortex that *knew,* left behind it a residue of nostalgia and guilt, which we mythologize as an expulsion from innocence. The human brain acts as the organ of knowing for the life process that began so long ago but, until humankind, did not know itself.

As the evolutionary biologist Bruce Weber put it in a conversation with me, "Much of the fear response is found [even] in the reptilian brain, since the high point of the reptilian brain is the amygdala and the limbic system. So although it is [later] fairly modified in mammals, and then in us, the basis is there early on.

"[In humans] , you still have that level which is almost nonreflective: an immediate reaction. At the biological level there is a feedback loop. You see something, and it gets processed in the brain and . . . is connected to potential danger. You are driving a car, and somebody swerves at you. You have this instant reaction. You see it, and your heart starts going.

"But then there is an additional level: self-consciousness, that 'autobiographical' consciousness. That's where you think: 'Oh, I nearly got hit by that truck.' And you think of things in the past. . . . That's where Damasio says you start getting your feelings, and they connect to sorrow. . . ."

I asked him if he agreed that all the fundamental emotions—that unconscious layer—are linked to physiological states.

"Damasio would say that all emotions are connected to physiological states," he answered. "The 'feelings,' then, are the conscious mind interacting with those emotions. The feelings are the mind contemplating the emotional state. Not that the mind is anything separate from the body. It's just that self-awareness, that autobiographical sense, is something that adds a dimension to what humans have.

"A cat has the 'emotions' and all of the physiological responses. The cat can be in the moment, but the cat is probably not aware that 'two years ago, I had a similar moment to this one.' The cat doesn't say, 'I really love playing with this ball of string, but someday I'll be dead and I won't be able to play with this ball of string anymore.'"

The brain, rather than being an organ with one function in the sense that the heart, lungs, and kidneys are organs, is instead the hub of communications for the entire organism, containing within itself a host of tiny internal chambers and structures, mini-"organs," in a way, some shaped like nothing found anywhere else in nature. Indeed the brain is the one organ that cannot be replaced and without which there is no life, no person. Though the human brain is probably unique, among earthly brains, in being able to examine itself, even the brain of a frog is a discrete "thing" only in a special sense of the word "thing"; it is a magical "thing" that perceives.

From my reading I learned that the brain sits snugly and well protected within the skull, surrounded by a "tough fibrous sac" and "cushioned" by cerebrospinal fluid. Its most striking structural feature is that it comprises two roughly symmetrical halves, the right and left hemispheres. These are linked by a strip called the corpus callosum ("tough body") and joined to the spinal cord, which stretches down through the vertebrae of the back. Small threads of nerve bundles travel down the spinal cord, connecting the brain to the rest of the body. The two hemispheres of the brain are far from identical in function, the right hemisphere being famously more emotional, intuitive, and sensitive than the more analytic and linguistic left, yet they mirror each other, observing the bilateral symmetry of our outer bodies. The bilateral symmetry of the brain goes back as far as the advent of bilateral symmetry occuring in animals more than five hundred million years ago.

Every internal brain structure comes in twos, except for the pineal gland at the "center, base of the brain," leading Descartes to hypothesize that the pineal gland might be the conduit between the brain and the feeling, thinking, immaterial "mind." The one extension of the brain that projects beyond the skull is the lining of nerves at the back of the eye that ophthalmologists can see when they shine a light into the cornea, the retina. Perhaps this is why we refer to the eyes as the "windows of the soul."

Though it weighs only three pounds, the human brain is, in Bruce Weber's words, "the most complex structure in the universe." While a heart might be plausibly likened to a pump, no model in the world as we know it—most emphatically including a computer—is analogous to the brain. The brain occupies an interactive relationship with the entire organism and between most of its own activities; it radiates outward beyond the body, monitoring and evaluating the immediate environment in which the body finds itself and, through thought and communication, with as much of the universe as it can take in. Through social life and language the brain is interactive with other brains; through nonverbal experience it connects with other creatures, with nature, with the ineffable.

When examined at the cellular level, the brain reveals neurons (nerve cells) of many different shapes and types serving different functions, but falling into three basic categories: those that send out information (efferent), those that receive information (afferent), and, by far the most numerous, the interneurons, which communicate between the two. The cell bodies of the neurons, when clustered together, create the dark portions of the brain, the "gray matter." These send out tubular connecting nerve fibers (axons) and branchlike dendrites, putting them in touch with each other and with the entire body by way of the spinal cord; these constitute the "white matter" of the brain. One axon can have as many as one thousand "terminals" in other neurons or in muscles as far away from the brain as the feet. The spaces across which nerve cells spark the electrical or metabolic activity of other nerve cells are called synapses, which means "junctures." Apparently there are roughly one hundred quadrillion synapses in the central nervous system. The electric signals sent by nerve cells may spark more such signals in other nerve cells, contraction in muscle cells, or secretions in gland cells.

From an anatomical point of view, the nervous system has

two branches: the central nervous system (the brain and spinal cord) and the peripheral nervous system (the network of nerves which extend from the brain and the spinal cord to the muscles, glands, and organs of the rest of the body). The central nervous system begins in the brain and through a web of connections flows down the spinal cord, initiating, monitoring, and responding to events throughout the peripheral nervous system. From a functional point of view, the nervous system operates in two ways: The somatic nervous system responds to our will and makes us conscious of our sensations, and the autonomic nervous system automatically and, for the most part, involuntarily, regulates our basic bodily functions.

Within the autonomic nervous system, operating primarily beneath the threshold of consciousness, are the sympathetic nervous system, which is primarily responsible for the release of energy, and the parasympathetic nervous system, which generally acts to restore equilibrium and coordinate the quiet buildup of energy. These two systems act in tandem, as linked and mutually necessary as the expansions and contractions of an accordion, regulating such activities as the operation of the heart and circulatory system, the lungs, the eyes, the salivary glands, the digestive system, the sweat glands, and erection of hair on the skin, the reproductive processes, the functioning of the liver, gallbladder, and kidneys.

We don't "choose" to be afraid. It is the sympathetic nervous system, triggered by the inner brain's instructions, that manufactures the physiology of anxiety and fear.

Infants are born with brains still in formation. At birth the limbic system, which constitutes much of what creates the "mental life" of birds, fish, and reptiles, is "much closer to fully formed" than is the "thinking" brain, and it continues to develop much more quickly than the uniquely "human" hippocampus and neocortex, which are associated with narrative memory and rational thought. It is believed that the amygdala, the almond-shaped "cluster of interconnected structures" found in both hemispheres of the brain in the limbic ring just above the brain stem (the word "limbic" comes from the Latin *limbus* ["fringe"]) and "responsible for the detection of potential threats" and for the "mobilization of defensive responses," is already operative at birth. The actions of the frontal lobes that allow the baby to comprehend and control the drives originating there only slowly begin to function at about six months.

The amygdala also stores the preverbal emotional information of early life. And for the remainder of our lives, it maintains a special role as a memory bank for our most intense experiences, because intense excitement and memory are chemically linked. The release of the hormones epinephrine and norepinephrine (synonyms for adrenaline and noradrenaline), which occurs during excitement (good or bad), starts from operations in the amygdala and circles back to it. When they return to the amygdala, these very same hormones trigger responses that enhance memory for moments of urgency. Normally impressions need to be reinforced by a kind of repeated reference before they become part of one's long-term memory. But nature has arranged for intensity to leave a lasting imprint. The visceral impact of a moment of ecstasy or horror can be burned into the brain in a moment in a way that makes its later recollection unusually primitive.

When emergencies occur in early childhood, they are therefore preserved in a kind of physical memory, so that they can serve as useful guides for future behavior. Early encounters with pain—being burned by touching a flame, for example—are preserved in one-time learning. Such preverbal memories forever retain the power and mystery of the stage of brain development at which they were formed. It is not until roughly the age of three that the hippocampus in the limbic system begins to store longer-term memories. Therefore Freud's view that the first five years are the crucial ones in determining personality, even while much of what occurred then remains permanently hidden from consciousness, is compatible with our current understanding of brain development. Events during that time leave their fingerprints on the wet clay of the coalescing mind. According to anxiety authority Dr. David Barlow, experiences of extreme stress, such as a separation from the mother, experienced in early life, create "permanent alterations in brain function" that make one particularly susceptible to depression and "chronic anxiety" later on.

While the brain of a child is particularly malleable, even having the ability to duplicate the functions of two hemispheres in one, if one hemisphere is irreparably damaged, the brain continues learning and reforming itself throughout life. Whatever is perceived as helpful to future survival (again, for good or ill) is likely to be neurally preserved. Neurologist Gerald Edelman refers to this as the Darwinism of the synapses. In a sense, then, there is no firm dividing line between experience and brain chemistry. Experiences and behaviors create and strengthen neuronal connections. Even in crustaceans, whatever happens leaves a mark on the subsequent chemical makeup of the brain. In studies of crayfish, for example, it has been demonstrated that neurotransmitters in the brain have "different effects" on the release of serotonin depending upon "the previous psychosocial experience of the organism." Just as often happens in people, those in charge feel better, become more confident, and therefore are more likely to stay on top. In other words, social dominance or subservience in these crustaceans seems to alter their very brain structures, contributing to their bullish mood and to the perpetuation of their status. Yet these brain effects can still be reversed if their experience changes (i.e., if another fish takes over). As Oliver Sacks puts it, "Instead of seeing the brain as rigid, fixed in mode, programmed like a computer, there is now a much more biological and powerful notion of 'experiential selection,' of experience literally shaping the connectivity and function of the brain (within genetic, anatomical, and physiological limits, of course.)" It is therefore no mere figure of speech to say that what happens to us becomes a part of us. Just as our faces, our hands, our skins, our hearts, and our lungs reflect our habits, so do our brains. In other words, what we do, feel, and live through is what we become.

Originally the brain was considered to operate as a whole. Even Hippocrates (ca. 460–ca. 377 B.C.), who identified with remarkable precision many of the brain's myriad functions, still considered that when the brain was unhealthy, it was due to its having been altered as an entire entity, by becoming, for example, "abnormally hot, cold, moist, or dry. . . ." (He associated a moist brain with madness.) The hypothesis that the brain contained localized sites for specific abilities and functions first proposed by phrenologist Franz Joseph Gall around 1800, and demonstrated experimentally by Pierre Flourens in 1825, was not fully confirmed until the early 1860s, when Paul Broca demonstrated that an injury to an area of the frontal lobe in the brain's left hemisphere caused a loss of speech. Later it was demonstrated that while many brain systems are duplicative and collaborative, with complex cross connections between the right and left hemispheres and between different areas within them, the human language system was to be found almost entirely in the left hemisphere. However, within this region, linguistic abilities turned out to be further separated. Damage to Wernicke's area (named for German neurologist Carl Wernicke) in the temporal lobe on the left side near the auditory cortex leaves people able to speak physically without being able to comprehend speech. An injury to the angular gyrus in the left hemisphere near the visual cortex impairs the capacity to read and write, while leaving the faculty of speech intact.

The perception of most of the senses is squarely bilateral, with the left hemisphere controlling and receiving all the senses and activities of the right side of the body, and the right hemisphere those of the left. (This mirroring is created by a crosshatching of nerve fibers inside the brain, as in a cat's cradle.) The exception to this is the sense of smell, which is monitored in the brain on the same side on which it enters. Some other brain capacities are centered more in one hemisphere than in the other, but with this activity shadowed in the same location on the opposite side.

The motions of our muscles are controlled primarily by motor strips in each hemisphere, which control motion in the opposite side. Thus, our right hand obeys our left brain, and vice versa. Our perceptions of what is happening in these same areas are relayed from sensory receptor cells throughout the body to somatosensory areas positioned immediately below these motor strips. The exact places where each muscle is directed and perceived have long been mapped. By far the most space in these motor strips is dedicated to the lips, the hands, the feet, and the genitals.

The distribution of functions in specific locations throughout the brain makes sense of the compartmentalization of activities we notice every day in the normal and so-called abnormal alike: in the autistic boy who can draw wonderful cartoons but can barely speak or in the scientist with outsize conceptual and mathematical skills but poor social skills.

Apart from those stored in the amygdala, long-term memories are apparently backed up in both hemispheres, "filed," as it were, at least twice. For this reason one can lose the workings of an entire hemisphere and still, thankfully, have access to much of one's past. In addition, memories form a complex system of cross-referencing based on sensory impressions. We know this firsthand when the sound of a melody reminds us of old love or the brush of warm summer air across the hairs on our arm bring on thoughts of a childhood friend. Not surprisingly, then, a far-off rumble of thunder can stir memories of an angry low voice or of the growl of a lion.

Recent studies of the brain have found exact locations for the activation of many of our subtlest activities, such as the recognition or interpretation of faces, the ability to orient ourselves in space, the ability to retrieve names for common objects, the ability to grasp large visual patterns, the ability to grasp detail, etc. Many types of general deterioration caused by diseases in the brain are now also well understood, even if ways of reversing them often remain elusive. For example, the progressive symptoms of multiple sclerosis—difficulties in vision, speech, and coordination—stem from an illness attacking the insulating myelin sheaths that protect and facilitate the workings of the neural axons, the circuits of brain communication.

The brain has been mapped in increasing detail in our time, but also with an ever-expanding appreciation of the extraordinary interconnectedness of its functions. While brain locations associated with surprisingly specific behaviors and experiences have been found, ranging from laughter to intention, even to spiritual ecstasy, there is also considerable caution about adopting a simplistic view of any of these mental phenomena. Most human character traits—a sense of humor, for example, or a sense of moral responsibility—require the interaction of so many facets of both hemispheres working in dialogue with each other that they constitute a symphony of almost infinite complexity. According to Oliver Sacks, even "a single conscious visual percept" may "entail the parallel and mutually influencing activities of billions of nerve cells."

The fear response is something admirable. Those of us who are subject to its misfiring shouldn't blame the response itself. Every single ingredient in it is the result of millennia of adaptations that helped creatures survive.

A fear response is triggered by the brain's deduction that it should mobilize the body for danger. What were the dangers when Neanderthal and *Homo erectus* and the early *Homo sapiens* lived on our earth? Perils included not only the predators but all places from which escape from predators and natural disasters would be difficult or where one would be particularly vulnerable to assault. These would include territories at the heart of many of our modern fears: open spaces where there is no place to hide; caves and closed-in spaces where danger could be concealed or where we might be trapped; the dark, where visibility and mobility are denied us; heights from which we could not save ourselves; in fact, any unknown terrain where ignorance would put us at a disadvantage. To an early hominid, alert to risk, fear could strike at a loud noise, which might signal a hostile presence or natural calamity; at a loud voice, signaling an angry superior; or even at the failure to perform an expected task, which could result in his being ostracized.

It is logical to assume that our hominid ancestors also had fears that simply came from within—when they were sick, when they were in the dark or alone, or when they had disturbing dreams. In addition, some of them must have been subject to the genetic flaws that cause excessive fear and anxiety today. Such people could not but take their fears seriously. Since an association between fear and danger is simply hardwired, they must have taken their fears to be omens of danger that they alone received.

Chapter Five

Fear

I am well aware that I am no more qualified to discuss the workings of the human brain than I am to dance the role of the prince in the ballet *Sleeping Beauty*. Yet in order to understand my own limitations, which so often seem at odds with the very things I want to be doing, I have had to try to grasp something about the way the brain protects and facilitates our existence by coordinating our reactions and behavior, to understand something about fear, and to contemplate the fact that, in its complexity, the human brain can instigate a fear reaction for a variety of reasons.

The primal emotions, in Damasio's sense of the term, are designed to "move" us. When such emotions are possessed by creatures with a human mind, they lead to complexities entirely new in nature. Though our fellow animals also carry within them the mechanisms for tidal surges of impulse and feeling their brains do not, as far as we know, interpret these responses in metaphorical ways. In humans these physiological mechanisms lead to interplays of the physical and mental, generating art and rituals and myths and love and hate and warfare. The brain also makes use of the body's physiology for its own ends, interpreting the body's language and the world in unexpected ways. In humans, survival mechanisms like fear can be turned into a handicap; necessary appetites can become life-threatening compulsions; aspects of intelligence can be turned into self-destructive obsessions; the body's protective immune responses can mimic organic physical illness.

A cockroach exhibits a fear response fleeing from danger with frantic energy, using every ounce of strength to climb from the sink as it fills with water. Yet it is not believed that a cockroach has what we would call consciousness. In fact it is suspected, although no one can say for sure, that even in those animals closest in consciousness to us humans, the foreknowledge of death is absent, even where there is the instinctive fight to survive. The experience of threat instills terror and a fight–flight response, but without what humans would call knowledge.

I asked biologist Betsy Sherman when she thought our human sense of anxiety emerged and if she thought that phobias were unique to humans.

"I do think that nonhumans share something that we would all recognize as anxiety," she told me. "Whether chimpanzees have bizarre fears of rocks of a certain color, say, I don't know. But I certainly think that they understand anxiety, even anxiety in social circumstances. They have an amygdala. And as a character in a Michael Ondaatje novel says about the amygdala: 'It houses fear and therefore governs everything.'

"Back in the day, when we were being chased by a cave lion, our heart rate would go up, all of that autonomic stuff would happen, and we would either climb a tree and escape or we were eaten. In such circumstances that fight-or-flight reaction would settle down after a while, once the threat was gone.

"The conventional wisdom is that we transplanted this same reaction to the modern world, where our boss is screaming at us, or we are worrying about paying the rent, and that the triggers for that response [fight-or-flight] persist, even though it originally evolved in a situation where it wasn't meant to be a chronic response.

"But my take on it is that we were living in the equivalent of Siberia back in the day, and in the winter we all were in the same cave together—mothers and sons and daughters, cousins, uncles and aunts. I think there must have been persistent anxiety in early humans, just anxiety about social relations, that might have turned on these very ancient responses. So I think that the displacement of this fight-or-flight response predates modernity. I think that we were anxious for all the time we've been human."

She took a deep breath and continued. "We have this cortex, this new thing, and we rationalize [our emotions], but the [emotions] themselves are old and deep.

"I don't know how old phobias are. I don't know if you need a neocortex to have a phobia. But I bet you do. Phobias would be part of the cost-benefit equation of having this vast new part of the brain. Part of what comes with knowing."

What we call fear (the "phobos" in "phobia") is a type of arousal, physical and psychological, that spurs action in an emergency. Darwin's description of fear corresponds to the physical effects initiated by this arousal, which begins in the brain and is carried out by the autonomic nervous system. Fear, like pain, is unpleasant and, like pain, necessary.

What sparks the amygdala and nervous system into action and makes us afraid can be an idea or memory (conscious or unconscious), a sensory impression (a sound, sight, smell, or touch), or an internal physical sensation (such as palpitations or pain). In fact some of us are so sensitive to our own sensations that we can overreact to our bodies' signals (anxiety sensitivity). Much study has been done on the subject of such introceptive conditioning, which helps explain how the fear system can be mobilized by imperceptible physical symptoms, which are then mistakenly interpreted as a threat to the organism.

For the same reasons, anxiety reactions to heights, open spaces, enclosed spaces, water, the dark, and loud noises can sometimes originate in an oversensitivity to the physiological changes these situations cause, rather than to their "symbolic" import. (Panic at being at a great height does not necessarily stem from fear of success!)

The mind responds by association. Things rustling underfoot, something looming overhead, a suspicious, noxious smell, chemicals of rage rising in a creature standing in front of you— these things stir our memories. Is this a problem? What happened last time? Is this a cue to move away?

How do we know when to cope with danger? Ordinarily our senses relay most information to the butterfly-shaped thalamus. This in turn sends its impulses to the neocortex, where the right and left prefrontal lobes, holding each other in balance, analyze and coordinate emotional and behavioral responses. In his book *Emotional Intelligence,* Daniel Goleman describes the left prefrontal lobe as almost like a "neural thermostat," moderating the aggressive and fearful responses of the right prefrontal lobe. That these prefrontal lobes house much of what makes for emotional experience and interpretation is borne out by the flattening effects prefrontal lobotomies had on mental patients and criminals.

Considering the bewildering complexity of all the information we are faced with, this evaluative system is surprisingly reliable. In dangerous circumstances like the one I faced that Halloween night in 1975, the brain springs into action instantaneously. The frontal lobes quickly direct the amygdala to trigger the autonomic nervous system to initiate a fight-or-flight response. However, as mentioned in the previous chapter, there is also a shortcut for emergencies. The work of neuroscientist Joseph LeDoux demonstrated that a small neural pathway proceeding directly from the thalamus to the amygdala *before* passing through the neocortex constitutes a kind of express road to emotional activation. This bypass gives the chemistry of fear a head start over thought processes. In situations where one has no time to think, the speed of this physical reaction can save one's life. But in those for whom fear comes too easily, it may activate a feeling of terror without giving them the time to sort out what is happening.

It is important to remember that without the amygdala and its ability to help us protect ourselves, we would have become extinct long ago. People who suffer from damage to the portion of the amygdala connected to the fear response (a rare consequence of illnesses, such as Urbach-Wiethe disease, that are associated with calcium deposits in the brain) lose the ability to defend themselves, sense danger, look afraid, or even recognize threatening expressions in others. They lose the very concept of fear.

When the amygdala sends its alarm signals, the sympathetic branch of the autonomic nervous system goes into action. Naturally the system might sense a need momentarily, causing a brief spike in anxiety, only to shut off just as quickly. But it is exquisitely sensitive to the moment by moment changes in our inner and outer weather. While its alter ego, the parasympathetic system, has a calibrated, selective, and nuanced effect on its terrain, the sympathetic system tends to act as a whole and all at once.

After causing adrenaline and noradrenaline to be released from the adrenal glands, making it possible for the emergency response to sustain itself, the autonomic nervous system fosters preparedness for action. Heart rate, strength of heartbeat, and blood pressure increase, rushing oxygenated blood to the major muscle groups, such as the legs and the heart itself, which will need extra power if one is to run or put up a fight. The rapid heart rate (sometimes including palpitations) is more than perceptible, and the power of the heart can sometimes be felt like a drum in one's chest. In the process, blood flow is redirected away from the face, skin, fingers, and toes. This acts as a protection against bleeding and causes pallor in the face and sensations of coldness, tingling, or numbness in the feet and hands. When the response is first activated, one can feel a flash of bodily heat as the nervous system is awakened, followed by a sudden coldness as circulation flows from one's extremities.

At the same time breathing becomes deeper and quicker, bringing in more oxygen to the lungs to be pumped to the muscle tissues. The adaptive purpose of this is to increase one's strength. In the event of actual flight or physical action, the body uses up this extra oxygen at the rate it is taken in. However, in an anxiety attack it constitutes overbreathing (hyperventilation), which causes a decrease in the amount of carbon dioxide in the blood and a rise in its alkalinity. This can cause sensations of choking or smothering even though one is in fact breathing very effectively. Emily Dickinson captured the experience in this strange, halting poem:

> I breathed enough to take the Trick—
> And now, removed from Air—
> I simulate the Breath, so well—
> That One, to be quite sure—
>
> The Lungs are stirless—must descend
> Among the Cunning Cells—
> And touch the Pantomime-Himself,
> How numb, the Bellows feels!

The sudden strenuous breathing also fatigues the muscles in the chest wall, causing sensations of tightening in the chest and sometimes chest pain. Naturally such symptoms, if mistaken for heart attack, are in themselves frightening.

During this inner exertion the sweat glands become activated to moderate body temperature, generating an outer slipperiness that may have once hindered attackers in the wild. This can cause a sensation of being both hot and cold simultaneously, since the exertion of hyperventilation and the stepped-up energy production occurring inside heat up the body, while the flow of blood away from the skin and the increased outer perspiration cool it.

The response in the digestive system is also paradoxical. On the one hand, it rushes to purge itself, increasing mobility, and possibly also acting as protection against becoming appetizing to predators. However, at the same time, blood and energy are also directed away from the digestive system to where they are most needed, causing the activity in the gastrointestinal tract to shut down, bringing with it nausea and intestinal discomfort. This slowing of the digestive functions carries with it a decrease in salivation, producing thirst and dry mouth and making swallowing more labored. It can also give one choking sensations. In the process, throat muscles sometimes constrict with tension, which, along with the decrease in salivation, causes the voice to become hoarse or strained. There is no advantage to having a pinched voice when one is frightened. As Bruce Weber explained to me, when natural selection selects for one factor—in this case, muscle tightening—other, superfluous effects often "come along for the ride."

Hyperventilation causes a constriction of blood vessels and brings about a temporary, minor, and harmless decrease of blood flow and oxygen to parts of the brain. This can contribute to feelings of confusion, dizziness, and light-headedness and cause transient blurred vision. It is part of what causes us to say in anxious circumstances, "I can't think straight." Additional visual symptoms can result from the dilation of the pupils, which widen to allow in more light and extend peripheral vision.

None of this is actually harmful and in fact can be countered voluntarily with breathing exercises.

Another common symptom of fear is visible in animals when they are trapped; the freezing response known as tonic immobility. In addition to fighting back or fleeing, the option in the face of danger is to remain quiet enough to evade detection, to quell the instinct for predation in creatures that pursue only animals on the run. Feigning death can save an animal's life, and in some creatures the feigning mechanism is instinctive. In humans the first response to an ominous noise or sight is often to become as still as possible. In such a state one is alert to every sound and motion; one becomes pure perception. In fear we often experience more than a trace of this, with sensations of stiffness and rigidity. The experience is universal enough for the phrase "scared stiff" to require no explanation. Rape victims sometimes report having experienced an extreme version of this, a trancelike, quasi-paralytic state during the attack, in which they feel cold, numb, and impervious to pain, even though they are fully conscious of what is occurring.

Our faculties of attention are uncannily mobile and complex. The regulation of awareness, which we experience as voluntary, is naturally only partially so. This becomes obvious if we think of how much information bombards our five senses at a given moment. The act of directing our attention to things requires a host of mental receiving and sorting mechanisms that are coordinated by the reticular formation, a section of the brain running through the brain stem. In fact this center for attention is not fully developed until puberty, helping account for the short attention spans of childhood.

Much of the time our attention is divided among a host of things, infinitely more information than we could possibly process consciously. For the most part we keep many different levels of attention in a hierarchy. Just think of how football players monitor every member of the opposing teams or the way nursery school teachers keeps track of a roomful of children, with an additional eye out for the troubled child or the child who has been sick. Just as we have peripheral vision, we seem capable of peripheral attention.

Strong emotion focuses the attention on one thing, holding the rest of the intellect hostage. The grip of this focusing mechanism and the degree to which it blots out other mental concerns vary according to need. Danger galvanizes the mind. When we are afraid, just as our blood is concentrated in the major muscle groups essential to a strong response, so the energies of the mind become concentrated on a threatening object. This is analogous to the way pain can direct our attention to an injured place in our body. A line from W. H. Auden comes to mind: "For who when healthy can become a foot?"

How often have you suddenly found that the presence of something disturbing (like the bat that once flew around my head during a concert performance I was giving) became at first distracting, and then, oddly, *all* you were paying attention to? The phenomenon, which can make even a tiny creature seem huge and menacing, is called macropsia. While indispensable in situations where one needs to direct all of one's attention to a threat, this same hyper-focus is inconvenient when applied to a mouse or harmless spider or an elevator or a bridge.

Oddly, the psychology of fear can also cause the illusion that the world is shrinking (micropsia). Dickinson seems to suggest both vertigo and micropsia in these lines:

> The earth reversed her Hemispheres—
> I touched the Universe—
>
> And back it slid—and I alone—
> A speck upon a ball—
> Went out upon Circumference—

After traumatic experiences people often report that they watched themselves as if from a distance, as if dreaming, as if what was happening were an illusion. The slowing of blood flow to the brain occurring in the body's response to danger can indeed contribute to mild dissociative symptoms: a transient sense of derealization, the sense that what is happening is unreal, and depersonalization, the feeling that one is detached from oneself. The inability to loosen one's attentive grip on the object of dread contributes to the sense of unreality, as extraneous thoughts are shunted aside. The environment even takes on a dreamlike shimmer as one's pupils enlarge to take in as much light as possible.

The protective usefulness of a state of detachment in an emergency is obvious, and transient experiences of depersonalization and derealization are normal and even familiar. These mental states pass almost unnoticed in moments of crisis. But when they appear seemingly unbidden and for no apparent reason, or in response to some eccentric dread, and are combined with the other symptoms associated with acute anxiety, they are profoundly unnerving. The phobic does well to remind himself at such moments that he is simply encountering the psychology of fear at an inopportune time, and that he is no more prone to psychotic states or to the more extreme forms of dissociation, such as dissociation identity disorder (multiple personality disorder) or fugue states, than is the next person.

In a state of high anxiety I have often felt this frightening loss of self, or, in the words of Maryanne Garbowsky, "strange, altered in some way" as if "on the edge of madness." Because of my own terror of mental illness and of the repercussions of displaying signs of it to friends and family, I am particularly unnerved by this symptom.

Since, as mentioned in the previous chapter, memories are "filed" in multiple ways, according to associations and to the impressions registered in all the senses, the special attentiveness of fear can be stirred by smells or facial expressions or physical sensations or noises or by odd phenomena recalling past experiences of danger or by thought associations. An element from a remembered threat will rouse a readiness for fear. Our brain is constantly working, processing, comparing the present with the past, evaluating beneath the threshold of awareness. "Should I be wary because I was once mugged in a vestibule like the one I am in now?" "Ten years ago such a cracking sound above my head signaled that a heavy tree branch was about to fall on me. I had better look up and be prepared to run."

At the same time, the internal physical sensations associated with primary emotions open the memory banks for past experiences of those emotions. Physical sensations of rage stir memories of past anger. This is why the act of crying, even when formalized in mourning rituals, stirs sadness; why laughing, which stimulates a network of positive and relaxation responses, relieves pain by sending positive physical signals to our organs and muscles that contradict the negative ones. For this reason, then, the physiology of fear, which was created to mobilize us to face dire threats, also opens the memory banks associated with loss and desperation. Just as the triggering of an alarm system in a building sets hearts and minds racing, so the activation of our inner alarm system creates thoughts of doom, even when the original bodily stimulus is a harmless mouse or the mistaken impression that we are gravely ill (which Barlow would call a false alarm). Damasio reports upon a carefully controlled experiment in which subjects were called upon to move muscles in their faces in a certain order that, without their knowledge, simulated expressions of "happiness, sadness, and fear." Remarkably, by this purely mechanical means, the subjects experienced the moods associated with the expressions.

Conversely, memories and thoughts associated with the emotions stir their physical effects. If you imagine sorrowful events, you activate physiological sorrow. (Actors often have a gift for such autosuggestion.) This is why the imagination plays such an important role in abetting or allaying the physical symptoms of fear and indeed all the emotional states.

As I mentioned in chapter 1, a mind turned outward to true danger and hardship seems to loosen its grip on "manufactured" neurotic symptoms. "Legitimate" fear is ignited by danger and wanes when the danger wanes. By contrast, the phobic process is a continuous neurobiological loop that feeds only upon itself. It can be entered, as it were, at any point, increasing the activity of any part of the process. Dire thoughts and feelings fuel the neurological and physical events and are in turn inflamed by them. That is why an understanding of the fear process is deemed a component of cure. An analysis of the physical symptoms involved in the process and a restructuring of the thoughts that cause them, so that they are in line with external reality, can interrupt the fear cycle. There *is* after all a reality to be coped with: first, that one is having a phobic response to a situation that is, in and of itself, not dangerous; secondly, that the phobic response always runs its predictable course and, despite one's internal impressions, does not damage one's physical or mental health.

A mind that recognizes phobic fear symptoms, including the psychological effects, as distressing but benign, and that can address its own confusion and panicky feelings as parts of a natural process, can begin to tame a phobia. Otherwise, when the alarm bells of physical fear sound and there is no external danger, the brain becomes enmeshed in an absurd dialogue with itself:

"Hey! The alarms are ringing!"

"But it's just a drill, right? There is nothing wrong."

"Well . . . why else would the alarms be ringing?"

"I suppose because . . . you rang them."

"No, *you* rang them."

In fear, so pressing is the urge to run that sufferers of phobias rarely stay in a situation long enough to experience the complete chemical cycle in the presence of what they dread. The suppression of this inborn urge to flee is precisely what feels so distressing. It is in fact "going against nature" to resist it. While relaxation techniques and what the cognitive behaviorists call cognitive restructuring can mitigate or interrupt the cycle, the autonomic nervous system will do so regardless. The parasympathetic nervous system automatically restores normal blood flow and heart rate, counteracts hyperventilation, equalizes body temperature, relaxes the muscles, and creates the physical equilibrium associated by the thinking/feeling mind with safety. However, like fire trucks and police that hang around the scene of an accident long after the smoke has cleared, the sensations of tense alertness subside more slowly than they strike. This confirms their basis as a protective mechanism. After all, more predators could lurk where one has been spotted. The cycle ends when the chemicals of anxiety are fully reabsorbed by other chemicals in the body. If one is tired afterward, it is the natural fatigue after bodily tension and exertion. Like most physiological experiences, a panic attack can take many forms short of being full blown; it can exhibit only fragments from its complete repertoire of physical sensations.

Some evolutionists claim that our fears are holdovers from ancient times and that this accounts for the preponderance of phobias involving animals, heights, vast and enclosed spaces, the dark, and weather. Such phobias could then be seen as once-legitimate fears that might eventually wane as the human species continues to adapt to current experience. They might simply be old habits, no longer fitting the current world, like the tendency of urban dwellers who have moved to peaceful rural communities to continue to lock both their cars and front doors at night. Both Darwin and later Freud thought that, in particular, childhood fears were "phylogenetically endowed" remnants of outmoded protective responses. David Barlow points to strong evidence supporting the notion that at least two "behavioral fear systems" are evolutionarily primed: responses to predators and responses to those more dominant in the "social hierarchy."

There is ample evidence to show that fear can be contagious and strongly influenced by customs, stories, myths, plays, and movies. Some phobias are generated by traumatic incidents. Others may be connected to hidden symbolism or to troubling, often buried memories triggered by association. Many of us mimic phobias we saw in our parents or role models. The children of a friend of mine who is morbidly worried about germs have picked up his fear, complete with his habit of opening doors with a shirt or sweater sleeve so as to avoid contact with contaminated doorknobs.

While there is evidence of a whole range of genetic factors that might predispose someone to anxiety, panic, and phobia, it is also clear that these don't necessarily determine one's becoming phobic or how people will respond to phobic reactions if and when they occur. One can have a tendency to phobia without forming the habit of avoidance known as phobic behavior. In the same way, one can have a tendency to addiction and still resist becoming an addict. Traumatic incidents don't always result in phobias, nor does phobic behavior in a parent always instill the same in a child.

The genetic underpinnings of phobia have been the subject of much discussion but do not suggest any simple genetic path leading to the condition. In his majestic and comprehensive book *Anxiety and Its Disorders,* David Barlow cites research suggesting that anxiety and panic are not necessarily on the same continuum and may result from two distinct genetic predispositions. On the other hand, he proposes that in many people the two often interact; an inherited "proneness to anxiety associated with a biologically labile response to stress" may "interact with specific psychological and environmental triggers (internal and external) in a complex way to determine expression of fear and panic." To a layman like me this seems to mean that for many people the genetic predisposition is far from enough to determine a phobic personality. In studies of identical twins the results are confusing. A Norwegian investigation of identical twins found the risk of both's having panic disorder to be five times higher than the risk in a nonidentical twin control group. A similar Australian study seemed to point to a general inherited trait of "neuroticism" that was expressed differently in each twin, as obsessive-compulsive disorder, agoraphobia, or social phobia.

That anxiety, phobia, and panic run in families seems self-evident, but how specific and crucial is the genetic input is still not well understood. In describing the identification of a gene necessary for the transmission of serotonin in the brain, the chemical transporter 5-HTT, scientist Daniel Weinberger (of the National Institute of Mental Health) observed that genes having an adverse affect on mental health don't "make you sick in a vacuum [but help determine] how you deal with the environment." In the case of this one gene, for which there can be both long and short alleles, having two of the long alleles seems to correlate with the ability to withstand stress better. Even mice and monkeys with one or two of the short alleles of this gene show more fearful reactions when placed in stressful conditions, and humans lacking the long alleles exhibit "more intense brain reactions to fear stimuli" and a much higher incidence of depression following misfortune and stress than those with them. Thus, as I understand it, the lucky beneficiaries of the two long alleles can still be brought low by events but are genetically more likely to bounce back and face their fears, just as I can for a while, early in the morning, after a strong cup of coffee.

A reader of the *New York Times* "Science" section is confronted with a weekly announcement of newly discovered linkages between genes and personality traits, experiences and illnesses, physical ailments and psychological consequences, which are the subjects of claims and disputes and which generally turn out to be significant but not definitive. If even the merits of eating eggs is still being debated by dietitians, one can assume that the inner workings of human personality will not be indisputably explicated anytime soon. In sum, the fact that certain genetic traits "correlate" with particular character traits doesn't necessarily mean that they determine them.

Barlow summarizes the current understanding about the relationship between genetic inheritance and phobias: ". . . with our present knowledge, it would be difficult to assume that a specific clinical anxiety disorder—even a specific phobia—can be directly inherited as one intact behavioral and emotional response set in some sort of simple Mendelian mode, much as hair and eye color are inherited." But he also goes further and relates this to our current understanding of mental disorders generally: "At present . . . there is no behavioral or emotional disorder for which a classical Mendelian model of single-gene heredity seems applicable. Even for the major psychotic disorders, where genetic links have long been suspected, almost all investigators (including geneticists) believe that an underlying vulnerability interacts with a variety of psychological and social factors to produce the disorder."

There are several theories about which medical characteristics exacerbate phobias. The ear, the eye, the heart, and even responses to electromagnetic fields have been implicated in studies. Certainly anyone with phobic symptoms should see a doctor so that he can eliminate worries about underlying physical ailments.

There are also some convincing findings about which personality traits accompany phobias and agoraphobia. According to those who have observed hundreds or even thousands of cases like mine, phobics tend to be perfectionists, they tend to have an exaggerated need to please others, they tend to seek certainty, and most interesting of all, they tend to avoid showing certain kinds of emotion. The book *Your Phobia* has it that many of us have in common the "need and ability to present a relatively placid, untroubled appearance to others, while suffering extreme distress on the inside." This describes me rather well.

But if there is one indisputable fact that I have taken away from my own experiences and my readings, it is that a single psychological manifestation can result from multiple causes and can have multiple aspects. Even a symptom as discrete as a particular type of rash can reflect diet or allergy or experience or illness or many other factors. A phobia is clearly a constellation of interconnected components: physiology, thoughts, feelings, behavior. These enmeshed elements are not necessarily easily untangled. There is also the question of what positive role the phobia plays in a person's life. One might be using phobias for his own ends, even while trying desperately to get over them.

Chapter Six

Childhood

Driven frantically by this changing force,
I felt like a windmill in a tornado.
—TEMPLE GRANDIN

There was very little in my childhood home life to suggest that my father was not an excellent role model in almost all respects, and it seems logical to assume that I simply imitated his phobias, the way I imitated his sense of courtesy, or some of his speech patterns. But who actually serves as a child's role model, and in what ways, and for what reasons, is not a simple matter. Sometimes the apple falls so far from the tree that it lands on the other side of the earth. If children automatically picked up their parents' quirks, the neuroses of the world would be multiplying geometrically. And my brother would be exactly like me, which he isn't. (Although he does have some phobias, they are less severe and far less disruptive to his life than mine are.)

I had another model of behavior who not only was my sibling but had accompanied me in my journey into the world,

Mary, my twin sister. Mary was born five minutes before I was, in the early morning of August 27, 1948. We were six weeks premature, weighing roughly four pounds each, and we were kept in incubators for several weeks. In those days before sonograms or amniocentesis, twins were a surprise. At the time of the birth my father was home with a bad cold, and he and my brother received the astonishing news on the phone. My mother had been pregnant three times before: Before my brother, she had given birth to a baby girl who had lived only a single day; after my brother she had carried another boy for seven months and lost him in breech birth premature labor. My parents now suddenly had three children, and my brother must have faced the mixed feelings (excitement and devastation mingled) that an only child always faces when suddenly having to share his parents.

I—or, with respect to the dimness of early memory, the little boy I see in old photographs and home movies whom I know to be "I"—spent my first several years in the same room as Mary. Although it hardly seems possible, I remember with strange clarity being in a crib parallel to Mary's at the age of about two, rocking, while she quietly rocked back and forth alongside me. This was a nightly ritual, and I remember it as if it were I who echoed, or mirrored, her rocking. I can even recall the sensation I felt in the top of my head as it gently struck the headboard of my crib.

Mary was a delicate and beautiful girl, with an otherworldly quality. But she didn't smile at the age that smiling is expected, responded to voices slowly, was late to begin speaking, and was somewhat awkward in her coordination. In an old home movie taken when we were still in diapers, I can be seen doing a somersault that Mary tries and fails to imitate. My parents consulted specialists who suspected deafness, but this impairment was discounted, resulting in suspicions of some kind of autism. By the time we were two, it was increasingly evident that Mary was on a different track from her peer group. My parents began to differentiate between us more, and I believe that it was at that time that I began to sleep in my own room.

At age three and thereafter Mary began to be somewhat verbal, but her vocabulary and sentence structures were limited, and her speech was unusual, sometimes clipped and with a strange urgency, sometimes almost like singing. It was a noteworthy surprise whenever she initiated a thought or made an observation about something right in front of her. Once she looked out the window and said, "It's not snowing." More often she appeared to be remembering what had once been said, repeating remembered phrases that pertained to present occurrences, or speaking *sotto voce* to herself about what was happening. She could answer questions, but often the answers consisted of only one or two words. At the same time there was a very complex physical and nonverbal communication coming from her. She was fascinated by hands, her own and others'. Sometimes she would take one of my father's large hands palm up and study its lines for a long time. She looked at me with intensity, radiating an extraordinary emotionality and a kind of suppressed intelligence. I often had the impression that she was only pretending that she wasn't well. She looked as if she were holding back something enormous, some news that was not part of a child's world. There was a great pressure in her; sometimes you would see it in her eyes, and at other times it would just explode. Her eruptions were not just tantrums but a bursting forth of extreme inner distress. She would scream and kick and run through the house, sometimes holding her ears.

Like all siblings, Mary, my brother, and I achieved a kind of balance of temperaments in our play. We often did drawings, and Mary's remained abstract. While my brother was lively, brilliant, and humorous, with a tendency to "ham things up," and Mary delicate, volatile, and surrounded by a moat of mystery, I tended to occupy a more or less stable and apparently sunny middle ground. With Mary, I tended to be a kind of interpreter. This role carried over into school, where I was generally thought to have a good understanding of people. In first grade, when a Japanese girl spent the year in our class, I used to explain to the teacher what she was trying to say, and I believe that I was usually right. The Japanese girl and I became good friends, and she visited me at home several times.

If I acted up, it was probably mostly in relation to my brother. I was slavishly admiring of him and desperate for his attention. I would do almost anything to get a rise out of him, even if it resulted in his pummeling me. The most effective of my taunts was saying that he was "such a cute little baby." If I said this enough times in an unctuous, whining voice, he was eventually sure to reward me by chasing me down the hall and roughing me up. As an extra reward I could then complain to my mother, and she would chastise him for picking on someone so defenseless.

Mary did many things young girls do (or at least did in that era), such as play with dolls, but she did them in an exceptional way. She had a strange relationship to her arm, which she chewed, bit, sniffed, kissed, and talked to as if it were a friend. She in fact narrated her life to herself quite a bit, either repeating phrases about herself in the third person or speaking of things she hoped for. Sometimes her talking escalated, and its tone became fractious, as if two different voices were arguing within her. At times she looked beset by inner conflicts or anguished by physical pains that she wished would stop. Her movements seemed to alternate between being abrupt and being rather slow; nothing ever flowed, though she sometimes wore a look of great serenity and beauty.

She loved to listen to music and never tired of repeated listenings. Favorites were Broadway musicals like *Oklahoma!* and recordings of Maria Callas singing opera arias. She sang along, and amazingly, she could also pick the tunes out at the piano. She liked the mad scene from Donizetti's *Lucia di Lammermoor* sung by Joan Sutherland. She would often sing by herself at the top of her voice in her own special way. She also had her own sense of what was funny, and when she laughed, it would not be a social laugh, but an inward one as if she were being tickled. Sometimes I could make her smile with my drawings of funny faces, and she would look at the faces almost conspiratorially, as if they were real people, and grin from ear to ear.

In speaking to me about Mary, my parents kept their language as simple as possible, describing her as "slow." Their several attempts to place her in normal schools were failures. They explained that she was too difficult to handle and needed to be in a special place. At a certain point they began to say that she was retarded. Except when she was out of control, they seemed to see her as poignant, as a second "lost" baby girl. They loved her, but she stirred a terrible grief in them.

Sometimes I imagined that Mary suffered from hallucinations or heard disturbing sounds in her head. It is certainly likely that she had trouble sorting out competing stimuli and that many normal sights and sounds caused her pain. Autistic author Temple Grandin has described her own acute sensitivity to touch, sounds, odors, and activity and her difficulties processing it all as a child: "Various stimuli, insignificant to most people, created a full blown stress reaction in me. When the telephone rang or when I checked the mail, I'd have a 'stage fright' nerve attack. . . . Birthday parties . . . were torture for me. The confusion created by noise-makers suddenly going off startled me. The clamor of many voices, the different smells—perfume, cigars, damp wool caps or gloves—people moving about at different speeds, going in different directions, the constant noise and confusion, the constant touching, were overwhelming."

Lacking the normal brain's ability to listen selectively, Grandin could disregard an airport's chaotic bustle while reading but was unable to screen out the sonic background in order to speak comfortably on the phone. Noises of only moderate loudness made her hold her ears and scream. Even though she craved being hugged, normal affection made her panic. When she was agitated, spinning in circles or staring at a spinning top or coin helped her calm herself. She explains that the imbalanced nervous system of autistics makes them abhor some kinds of stimulation while craving those that relieve them of their inner turbulence. They apparently have a higher threshold for nystagmus, the flickering eye movements that, in concert with the vestibular apparatus in the inner ear, accompany our restoration of balance after we have spun around for too long. Autistics can often spend a long time spinning and, rather than become dizzy, find it soothing. In Grandin's account, they need relief from their inner state, and in order not to be overpowered by their senses and erupt in a tantrum, they "have to make a choice of either self-stimulating like spinning, mutilating themselves, or escap[ing] into their inner world to screen out outside stimuli."

My parents' attitude toward Mary reflected those of their milieu and time. My father was very tender with her and regarded her inner world, as he did everyone else's, with real respect, but he couldn't fathom her. My mother treated her as a daughter who simply stayed the same age while her sons matured. To both of them, I believe, she represented a form of innocence. Neither of them could take on the full-time task of attempting to decipher her experience on its own terms, to read into her own *way* of being a human being, or to discover her as their complete, if damaged, child.

Of course I sentimentalized her too. Even now I find her elusiveness, in some indefinable way, "magical." I don't often try to picture what the turmoil in her mind is like. I know that she wraps strings around her fingers until they endanger her circulation, bites and scratches herself, peels her fingertips and the skin below the fingernails until they bleed, and has a dangerous habit of stuffing string and plastic bags into her vagina. I know that she has at times been so intensely upset that she has needed to be restrained by more than one strong person. I remember her shrieks echoing through the halls of our apartment and the tormented energy of her crying, but I can't dwell on them for too long without trying to put them out of my mind.

With time she has lost the almost porcelain prettiness and look of utter normality that made it hard to believe that she was mentally and physically impaired. Of course she has been on medication for many years and that has taken its toll. But although she has now aged physically, in a way she has always seemed like someone who knows things that only an adult could know.

Mary is actually stuck at several developmental stages at the same time. She learned to write and spell to a first-grade level but can do any basic arithmetic problem without the slightest thought, by looking at it and providing the answer instantaneously. The same skill holds true for counting rows of items in a container: She can glance at the pattern and say immediately how many there are—even if the answer is as unexpected as "105." She can name the day of the week a holiday falls on years ahead. In her early teens she was taught to read music and memorized several pieces at the piano that she has never forgotten. If, in one of our rare reunions, I start to play one of them on the piano, she automatically jumps up and joins in alongside me, adjusting her tempo to mine.

Today she has retained most of her childhood patterns and in most ways has never become capable of leading what is considered an adult life. She seems to have an indestructible memory that makes few distinctions between past and present. Yet she can also integrate current changes into this picture. Told that our father had died, she connected the fact instantly with other people she had known who were "in heaven." She does not expect to see him again. She also took little time processing the fact that she had two new "relatives" (whatever that concept might represent for her) who were much younger than she (my two children).

Though Mary is more visibly "abnormal" than she was as a child, I tend to think of her as a sophisticated and richly textured middle-aged woman who happens to be strange and eccentric, someone who appears to be perceiving information carried over unusual wavelengths, who walks, acts, and speaks in an unusual way, rather than as "retarded." She exudes an essence of personality uncannily reminiscent of my father's and brother's. When I am with her, I feel a sense of wholeness, a kind of relaxation response. I often wonder what would have happened to her if she had been born into the—then rare—type of family that could have more resourcefully incorporated her into their routine.

Mary was undeniably my first romantic object. I can't remember my first three years, and I don't recall the cuddling, the intimate play of infancy, yet something makes me blush when I even try to remember it. Something in me pulls back in sadness from the thought of Mary's little face and delicate form and of the closeness that we lost. I remember our rocking alongside each other with a vague discomfort.

My own first explicit foray into sexuality, when I was six, was directed at a taciturn girl known for wildness and indecent exposure at school. It must reveal a Machiavellian streak in my nature that I invited her over to my house for the express purpose of suggesting an exchange of anatomical explorations. At least I was fair about it, proposing parity. But when we were discovered, naked, in my closet, I learned an unpleasant lesson about what was permissible. That is to say, the message I received from my father, who was deemed the appropriate person to arbitrate the matter later that same night, was ambiguous. "There is nothing wrong with what you did," he told me; "we just don't do it." In the confusion between his sense of post-Freudian enlightenment, his sense of fatherly responsibility, and his own convoluted circumspection, he forget to mention that six was simply a bit *early* to be doing it.

As a teenager I was almost phototropically drawn to girls who were quiet and hard to "read," who demanded some kind of special decoding in order to be understood. Although later on this became somewhat less the case, I continued to gravitate toward women who were, in some ways, "foreign" to the milieu of my childhood. The three primary relationships of my adult life have been with women born outside America, who were raised with unfamiliar customs and speak English with foreign accents. They all were from *somewhere else.*

I remember with a great wistfulness the atmosphere during my first eight years among Mary, me, and my dynamic, quick-witted, and already theatrical brother (at that time a devotee of magic tricks) despite the hidden pressures impinging upon us. My mother was intensely involved in the minutiae of our lives, generally cheerful and highly creative, but also high-strung and sometimes obviously overwhelmed by Mary's volatility.

There was also Bessie, an extraordinary woman who helped take care of the three of us, while doing most of the family cooking. She was from Virginia and had begun doing house-work and cooking after suffering from the nervous tension caused by working in a noisy factory. Her father, whom I later met at his ninetieth birthday, had grown up on a plantation as a slave. Bessie was childless and, as the years went by, increasingly directed her maternal feelings toward us. She played a crucial role in our childhood in countless ways, not the least of which was her matter-of-fact acceptance of Mary. As someone who had been on hand during the period of my brother's infancy and then for the birth of us twins and the unfolding of Mary's story, she helped support the entire apparatus of the family through the power of her acceptance of it. Mary was every bit as real to her as my brother and I were. Bessie was both extremely loving—her love also extended, however differently, to both of our parents—and somewhat dispassionate. Through being there (for what amounted in the end to forty years) to observe, make sarcastic asides, dispense advice, and remember the past, she helped reify the family.

She also could sometimes "handle" Mary in ways our mother could not. Mary was strong and fierce when she was upset. Her furies would erupt unexpectedly, even at a party, when she was dressed in a pink party dress and shiny black buckled dress shoes. Bessie was physically sturdy and could hold her when no one else could. Since she wasn't Mary's mother, she also wasn't frightened by her or by what her problems might signify.

Parents of a handicapped child often blame themselves and each other. After the initial diagnosis of autism—in that era deemed a "psychological" condition—was retracted, doctors studying Mary simply described her as retarded, a condition that had most likely been caused, they thought, by the circumstances of her birth. The "brain damage" could have been caused either by oxygen deprivation or by overoxygenation, both common occurrences in premature babies during that period. In more recent years, when I became responsible for reviewing and signing Mary's medical forms, I saw that she was listed both as "mildly retarded" and as suffering from "schizo-affective disorder."

I believe that my mother had always longed for a daughter. When she told me in later life about losing her first baby girl, she could not say the baby's name, Wendy, without conveying terrible grief. The loss was a wound that never healed. Throughout my childhood she held on to what remained of the family like someone carrying a precious package across a tampoon bridge straddling a ravine. Of course I didn't see it this way at the time. I merely thought that she seemed reluctant to let me grow up, sometimes almost hysterically overprotective, and that she needed to keep things in a kind of frozen permanence, as if the passage of time should be resisted. Perhaps from her perspective it did. When we had family arguments, they almost invariably revolved around whether or not my brother could do this or that activity that might be dangerous, too mature, or "overstimulating." In my case the disputes arose primarily when my brother proposed to take me along. Only rarely did I raise controversy on my own. I was already a turtle, and my head remained generally within my shell. In fact, when there were disputes, I got into the habit of taking notes on them, complete with descriptions of gestures and tone of voice, and then presenting a reading of them later to make everyone laugh.

My mother's father, a chemist, had died at the age of thirty-one, when she was three. The cause of his death, like so much else in our family history, may have been either deliberately concealed or remembered wrongly. His death certificate lists him as succumbing to tuberculosis, whereas my mother and aunt said that he died of work-related chemical poisoning. His name, like my father's, was William. As an infant my mother used to wait expectantly for him to return from work, and when he did, it was the high point of her day. She and her sister were raised by their mother, Rose, who worked for the postal service in Chicago. Rose never remarried.

My parents met when my mother was eighteen years old and already a reporter at the *Chicago Daily News*. My father's first cousin arranged the meeting, thinking my mother's vivacious, enterprising, and cheerful personality might do him good. The first encounter bowled him over, and he wrote in his diary that he had met his future wife. At that time she was forging ahead in the world, and her letters to my father, of which there are many hundreds, reveal a worldly, savvy, optimistic, and romantic young woman. They wrote to each other using pet names of the kind they continued to use up until my father's death, and during their early times of separation their near-daily communications were drenched in the poetry of mutual adoration and sexual attraction. They exchanged enthusiasms about writing and art, with my mother somewhat deferring to the range of my father's burgeoning intellectual interests. Although it took some months before she completely fell under his spell (she was a popular, ripely attractive girl, one year my father's senior), the two eventually became equally smitten, and by the time of their marriage, in 1929, they were famously inseparable, or "two against the world," as my mother's sister once put it.

When my parents met, they were intellectual equals, with

my mother being the tougher, more practical, and more experienced of the two. As a young woman she was not an unusually dependent person, and it was my father who appeared to be vulnerable and delicate. Their informal marriage ceremony, attended only by a handful of family members, was a declaration of independence for both of them. My father had turned twenty-one the day before and therefore could marry without parental permission. My mother wore what she pleased, a chic black dress. Both had been attending college, but had decided to leave. Their honeymoon was a nine-month trip to Europe, six months of which were spent in Paris, where my father worked every night playing the piano in a small club called La Cloche (The Clock). In Paris they made friends whom they knew for the rest of their lives. (One of them was the grandmother of my 1970s French girlfriend.)

In old pictures of my parents from the 1930s I am shocked by how good looking they are. My father looks like a diminutive Gregory Peck, and my mother is stunning and animated, with a dazzling smile. In contrast with my father, she was vivacious and sociable to her core, with an essential strength that never left her. In home movies from my early infancy she radiates confidence, and the camera, held by my brother, zooms in on her bright red lipstick. In the film of his fifth birthday party, right after my birth, she dances with him—at only five feet tall, she still towers above him—and he laughs angelically.

Something happened to her only a year or two later that is visible in these home movies, even when she appears for only a moment at the side of a frame. She looks shut down, tired and preoccupied, and, though still cheerful, as if she were no longer quite herself.

A change in her general state of mind during this period would certainly have been understandable. My father had become editor of the magazine, his romantic life had changed, and it had become apparent that one of their three children was mentally impaired. During this period she was in an automobile accident crossing Amsterdam Avenue and Ninety-seventh Street in a taxi, which left her with four broken ribs, cuts in her feet, and a pale-white four-inch crescent-shaped scar on the left side of her forehead where she had been struck by a flying piece of the driver's-side front window. I know that my father was as shaken by this accident as she was and that he related it, however irrationally, to her pain over his additional relationship.

But my mother's overall psychological history is mysterious. If she was delicately balanced, it showed mostly in her need to control and monitor things. She had the charming sense of command of a well-loved queen. Primarily cheerful, kind, and resilient, she could also become desperately alarmed and keyed up at times. At some point along the way she had abandoned her own aspirations and independence.

I know that when my father first left her in Chicago in the early 1930s to see what work he could find in New York, she became depressed. Later there were difficult years when they were first in New York together. While my father tried to write and compose, she found a number of fairly routine jobs—such as selling greeting cards—that never measured up to the glamorous one she had held at the *Chicago Daily News*, a job that she had managed to keep even during the layoffs of the Depression. A letter from my uncle to my father written about five years before her first pregnancy, in the late thirties, also suggests that she had a serious psychological setback during this period. In it he advises my father to be patient and not to expect the treatment of her problems to be an overnight success. Once my father's ground level job at "the magazine" worked out, she more than willingly abandoned any thought of a career for herself, and she never again thought of her intellect as being commensurate with his, or wanted to be viewed as a "career woman" (a phrase which she often preceded with the word "ambitious").

During my childhood my father's sexuality appeared to be under wraps—except when beautiful women appeared on television. By contrast my mother's references to sex were frequent and varied, veering between wistful anthems praising romance and pleasure and admonitions about the risks of hanging around "sophisticated" girls and the inherent dangers of being alone in a closed room with any member of the opposite sex, which seemed, in her view, to guarantee an eruption of passion. One of her favorite words in this context was "propinquity." She warned my brother and me against the irresistibility of sex by saying, "All it takes is propinquity."

Clinging steadfastly to her role of mother and wife, it seemed to distress her if her own interests, such as painting, were taken too seriously, as if that would destabilize things. Like many women of her day, I suppose, she considered putting on makeup before seeing anyone to be practically a religious commandment. She called this colorful mask her face, as in "I need to put my face on." When I was small, I was fascinated by the sophisticated and wonderfully hard-boiled look her features had when unadorned. To me, this highly intelligent, older-looking, more complex face was her real one, and I used to try to encourage her to leave off the makeup once in a while. She wouldn't. Her interest in journalism left a serious vestige in the form of her preoccupation with the news of the day. Indeed the degree to which matters of public concern occupied our entire family and dominated our family discussions can hardly be overstated. During the Vietnam War there was little else. During that period my mother would turn her chair around when President Johnson appeared on television, so she wouldn't have to look at him, since she held him responsible for starting the war.

In retrospect, it strikes me that my brother intuited that I needed to be looked after. He included me in his daily activities to a degree rare for a brother five years older. We played chess, checkers, Monopoly, Clue; we painted and drew, made home movies together, and put on puppet shows that explored the dark underbelly of life and tore the mask away from genteel society. In the home movies I followed his direction, cast either as his rival in deadly gang warfare or as the love interest.

Neither of us consciously knew that our parents were struggling with each other; there was too much evident harmony between them, and when we had breakfast in their bedroom in the mornings on weekends, there was an atmosphere of real coziness and family affection. There were times when our father's second ("office") phone would ring during these breakfasts and he would retreat with the phone into the closet. We didn't know that these were interruptions from his alternate life, but the oddness must have marked us anyway. Truth leaves a stain on things.

Any references to our father's finances remained unthinkable until after his death, at which point the shakiness of some of his arrangements was revealed, as was his inability to ask for the kind of salary he had deserved. He had needed, it turned out, to borrow extensively to shore up his various responsibilities, and at one point he owed loan repayments to no fewer than five different banks.

Even more submerged than the fact of my father's phobias were questions about my mother's mental health. Whether or not she had serious phobias I am still unable to say. She was apprehensive

about the weather to an unusual degree, referring to the possibility of a storm with the dread of someone from the Stone Age.
The fact that the weather was unpredictable and completely out
of her control seemed disquieting to her. She feared dogs, having had a bad experience with one as a child, and she warned us
of the presence of bees and wasps in a tone of serious alarm. She
couldn't and didn't drive, and she shared my father's need to direct every turn a driver should make while taking her somewhere. On the occasions when we traveled as a family in a
rented car with a driver, she held the map and dictated every
move. A drive to Lincoln Center was planned almost like a mil-
itary campaign. A taxi driver would be addressed with the utmost
courtesy but in a manner appropriate for someone who didn't
speak English, did not know the city well, and was hard of hearing. Neither of my parents would ever have dreamed of stating
the destination at the outset of the drive. The exact route was
doled out slowly, and the final destination always saved for last.
"Thank you. Now, we want to go down FIFTH AVENUE to
the EIGHTY-FIFTH STREET TRANSVERSE . . . and then
across to . . . COLUMBUS."

She maintained the same kind of firm grip in the kitchen,
and things that might have taken a half hour with some risks and
chances of a misstep could take an arduous two hours. Since she
kept close to my father, she never took a plane, and she never
took trips without him. I don't believe she was claustrophobic, but
I am not certain. She rode elevators with normal comfort, and
once when we were stuck in one together, she was calm, telling
me cheerfully that "the men" would come soon and let us out.
And yet she didn't take tunnels or subways when she was on her
own, any more than she did when with my father. Whatever her
own original fears might have been, her life gradually became
only marginally freer and more spontaneous than his, and her

sense of the world's dangers almost equally acute. After my father's death her patterns did not change. She never made the four-hour trip to visit me in Vermont, nor did she visit her sister in Arizona.

When it came to bringing me up, particularly in the wake of discovering Mary's condition, she applied her cautiousness to me with redoubled force. Although she often left me to my own devices, she usually specifically announced that I could do whatever I wanted to, as if without her permission, I might not feel able to. I was small and was frequently roughed up at school in my first years there. I have a distinct memory of playing on the school roof at age four or five and being pinned under a tire that a tough kid decided would make a nice impression on me. Nevertheless, according to a (very well-written) school report from 1954 that I found recently, I would "not let other children infringe too far" on my rights. "When someone tries to take the bicycle he is using away from him or some other prized possession, he puts up a courageous fight." Apparently at that time I was "always eager to try out a new experience whether it be cooking or going on an errand."

My mother encouraged me to stand up for myself, but she also kept a closer watch on what I did than on what my brother did, guarding me, delaying seemingly forever the moment when I would be allowed to cross the street by myself, and cultivating a sense that I wasn't ready to "handle" this or that activity, this or that scary scene in a movie. My memory is that as a child I developed, as it were, with the brakes on. Whether they were only my mother's or my own too, I can't be sure. I do remember her zero tolerance of risk. We were told to be wary of catching colds, and early-warning signs of colds were pounced upon. In cold weather we were bundled up, and our galoshes were never forgotten. I watched the green-faced witch played by Margaret

Hamilton in *The Wizard of Oz* through my mother's fingers, tightly pressed against my eyes lest I develop nightmares. I learned later of the many times she had called my teachers with worries about me. When I was ten, I used to visit my friend Hank, whose family had a house on a pond in Cape Cod, and I enjoyed taking the motorboat out into the middle of the pond by myself. When my mother called and heard that I couldn't come to the phone because I was out in the motorboat, her distress had a wildness, according to Hank's mother, that went beyond the cause. (Admittedly, I was a poor swimmer.) During one of my Cape Cod visits when I was around the same age, I was offered a ride on a private plane belonging to a friend of Hank's family, an orchestra conductor bearded like a member of the Three Musketeers, but my mother called to say that I could not go along.

I don't recall her being depressed—quite the contrary—but I do think that her ability to concentrate was compromised in her early middle age. Although she wrote long and flawless letters to us when we were away at school—always characterized by her impeccable spelling, grammar, and handwriting—retained old phone numbers and memories no matter how much time had passed since she had last thought of them, maintained a detailed grasp of current politics and social issues, and kept up with newspapers and with the magazine, she seemed to struggle when it came to reading a book of any length and spent long hours accomplishing small tasks. She didn't like to see people just sitting around doing absolutely nothing and abhorred the notion of wasting time. At the same time, while her own activities always had a goal, she would sometimes grow tired of focusing on what she was doing and be terribly unproductive. In the end, as mysterious as my father was, his history is clearer to me than my mother's. She had no confidantes, and she kept whatever pain she was feeling mainly to herself. Even her exact age remained a secret until she was almost ninety and the decline of her health necessitated my brother's and my intervention.

There was an across-the-board policy of secrecy about so many matters in our family that one almost required a special handbook to remember them all. There were many admonitions not to mention things publicly that were right under our noses and many deeper issues that remained buried or unmentionable. When I once raised the subject of our all being short, I was handed a long string of qualifiers and objections to my having put it precisely that way. (We *were* short.) When I referred to our family as, in its own quiet way, "competitive," there was a chorus of dissent and explanation. When I gave as evidence that our father never even *considered* that there could be better editors in the world than he was, there was a long silence. I had them there.

Being Jewish was also a matter for some distant uneasiness, at least enough for it to be fun for my brother to begin a dining table discussion, "Well, we Jews . . ." There was never any denial of being Jewish, but there were no relaxed assertions of it either, and the idea that it had a meaning was dismissed. This general subject is worthy of an entire book, of course. My parents weren't remotely religious, and their ties to ancestral customs meant nothing to them. Despite the fact that objectively, many of their character traits and habits could be seen as quintessentially Jewish, they belonged to a generation eager simply to be Americans. Their ambivalence made perfect sense, but it also shaded over into discomfort.

My father, along with one of his brothers, had changed his last name from one that could be mistaken for Chinese (Chon) to one that suggested that we might be Irish, or at least Anglo-Saxon. (The original Polish, Russian, or German name from which "Chon" derived has remained a mystery.) Mary's full name sounded still more Christian, and when she was referred to at her schools as Protestant, my mother made no objection. My father had a love of Jewish humor and would laugh as soon as Henny Youngman appeared on the TV screen or when someone started a joke "Two Jews were talking at a bar . . . ," but he seemed to distance himself from people who loudly proclaimed their Jewishness. Sometimes people do use their ethnicity as an easy way of establishing a sense of identity and to give themselves a false sense of belonging, an almost irritating pride in their background. My father was trying to establish himself as an independent citizen of the world, free from a constricting membership in this or that "clan" and with sympathy for humanity generally. On the other hand, there was some kind of revulsion there too. He seemed to shrink from identifying himself in any open way with a group that had been despised or with all those who had died because they were of the very background he shared. When a minister friend of my brother's visited the house and said a prayer at Thanksgiving dinner, he was deeply moved, but it is hard to picture him being as moved if the friend had been a rabbi.

My mother clung to a belief in her ancestors' strong Swedish connection and believed that her own mother, Rose, had been born in Karlstad, Sweden. Although my brother and I later confirmed that Rose had in fact been born in Russia and that her family had traveled—or, more probably, fled—to Sweden on their way to the United States when she was an infant, at exactly the moment that many Jewish families did the same thing (during the pogroms of the 1880s), it isn't clear where the myth originated: with our mother, our grandmother, or even our great-grandmother. What is clear is that it was preferable to be sentimental about the Swedish connection than to speculate about the Russian one. A suspicion lingers that an event of true horror, the violent death of my grandmother's twin baby sister, could have motivated this blurring of memory. Only recently could I ascertain that my grandmother kept kosher, and that my mother grew up lighting Sabbath candles and even grudgingly attending Saturday services with her older sister.

As children in New York City we celebrated a religiously deracinated Christmas and Easter, and I, like so many other boys of Jewish background, played shepherds and wise men in yearly Christmas pageants, gazing adoringly at the lightbulb representing the holy infant.

At least a small grain of the family habit of silence and secrecy can be traced to the remote European terror that left such a long shadow on so many Jews of the time, as persecution always does. It added one more layer of mystery to an already overburdened pile of mysteries in our childhood lore.

My parents had their hands full: with their marriage, with their secrets, with Mary, with their sons, with my father's double routine, with the relentless pressures of his job, with their strained finances, with the sadness they carried of two children who hadn't survived, and with their individual mental histories. As if by instinct, my brother and I created a microclimate of our own within the family. This protected me to a degree and helped me learn how to be someone other than just Mary's twin.

During my childhood my mother seemed to focus almost all her considerable strength and intellect on the minutiae of family life. Having voluntarily curtailed her own independence, she oversaw with rather extreme vigilance the circumscribed world in which her children grew up, all the while trusting that by virtue of our own travels and experiences at rustic summer camps and schools, we would learn to flourish in the wider world. While my father conveyed by his habits an aversion to all kinds of specific circumstances, my mother conveyed through her attention to immediate details a sense that the world beyond ours was almost out of reach, that we had to cling to the things that we knew. While, like many mothers of musical children of the time, she seemed to have a fantasy that I would one day lead a life as glamorous as Leonard Bernstein's, she feared the rebellions, aggressive self-assertions—the growing up—that achieving such a life would actually require. A different kind of person from me, or one who was not a twin with my early traumas, or someone with a different kind of mind or a different set of childhood experiences would simply have made his way from childhood to adulthood with the usual mix of rebellion and wistfulness. Instead, it would seem, I internalized her conflicted message and made it part of who I am.

Chapter Seven

On the Road

. . . A dog in extreme terror will throw himself down, howl, and void his excretions . . . with every muscle of his body trembling, with his heart palpitating so quickly that the beats could hardly be counted, and panting for breath with a widely open mouth, in the same manner as a terrified man does.
—CHARLES DARWIN

Mankind cannot bear too much reality.
—T. S. ELIOT

After almost twenty-five years of marriage, I was divorced in 2001. Naturally I hoped to experience companionship once again, but this necessitated sharing my problems with someone new. As a courtship strategy a declaration of agoraphobia would appear to be risky. Fortunately my new companion didn't mind the sound of my problem, but she was quite amazed when she first saw it manifested.

The truth is that I feel equally amazed. I have never felt that my phobia problem suited me, and it often surprises me. Despite being perpetually on guard, I sometimes walk into a phobic trap without thinking about it. My first coping mechanism when seized by the familiar symptoms of panic is to remind myself that I am in fact a phobic and that I tend to react this way. This already gives me some handle of objectivity on the true situation, which is not that I am in actual danger but that I have a pernicious learned response to many situations. Still, I remain dumbfounded at how automatic, instantaneous, and severe my reactions are, not to mention how trivial the triggers can be.

When I was first spending time with my new companion, I had difficulty walking down a road that was perhaps at most four-tenths of a mile long but was bounded on both sides by large open fields. She would accompany me in my attempts to walk the route. At either end were buildings, but along the way there was, in a sense "nothing."

I don't have too much trouble walking many miles at a time in busy New York City, but when I got halfway down this empty road, I would freeze in place and balk at continuing, exactly like a dog who freezes at the door to the veterinarian's office or a horse who refuses to walk over a rotten bridge. I couldn't be convinced that I could continue to walk despite whatever symptoms I felt and that if I did so, I would in fact get to the end of the road and still be the person I was four-tenths of a mile back. The physical reactions included my becoming short of breath and beginning to breathe rapidly (in fact to pant like a dog), feeling my heart beat at twice the normal rate, getting extremely warm and sweaty and feeling like discarding my coat and jacket, finding my vision growing dark and blurred, feeling my face grow cold, and my legs tremulous, weak, and then extraordinarily stiff. I oriented myself by seeing how far I had walked from one small tree to another, but at a certain point, less than halfway down the road, I would stop and simply wouldn't budge.

I couldn't seem to get past the point at which I would be closer to the destination than to the point of origin. Perhaps this mirrors the psychology of every experience in life. The midpoint of any journey is the point of maximum tension and isolation, the farthest distance from either end. The far end tends to be the unfamiliar one. The going is always metaphorically uphill; the return trip, downhill: tension and release. But being this sensitive to the process is beyond maladaptive; it's nuts!

I was convinced that when I reached the midpoint of the road, my legs would not move at all and that I would be trapped in place there. I had a vivid picture of myself standing at the center of emptiness, screaming. More recently I have read of those who have difficulty crossing a city street, and they too identify the fear that they will be frozen in place in between either corner, just where the cars need to pass.

I should mention that in order to undertake this tiny journey, I had come equipped with all my "safety items." I was wearing my jacket, which contained a paper bag—of the type I breathed into once, many years ago, to calm myself when I suffered a concussion—and a (largely unused) container of the anti-anxiety medication Xanax, and I carried a bag containing a bottle of ginger ale and my cell phone. Even a cursory look at these items, assembled seemingly at random, shows that they all relate directly to panic symptoms. The ginger ale—a stand-in for sustenance, generally, and perhaps even maternal comfort—helps relax the tightened throat and compensates for the dry mouth and pinched voice of fear; the tranquilizer rescues tense muscles, racing heart, and frantic mind; the paper bag restores breathing to a normal capacity; the cell phone contacts "help."

My friend was astonished. She tried to coax me, offered a kiss as a reward, promised not to leave me stranded. I wouldn't move. "Wow, you really can't do this," she said.

A month later I did do it, in fact, and what made the difference was actually simple. It had been explained to me that the freezing response was part of the physical repertoire of fear and did not constitute true immobility. Once I had grasped that this sensation was not something peculiar to me but was merely one of the muscular results of the fight-or-flight response, which (I now learned) is also sometimes called the fight-flight-*freeze* response, I mustered the trust in my own ability to continue walking to get to the end of the road. I still carried my cell phone and panted like a dog, but I succeeded. Since then the walk has become easy, and I can do it without carrying anything.

If you are very attuned to sensations in your legs, you will notice that they seem to have a mind of their own. They may twinge when you look up at a tall building or look down from one, they tighten instantly when you are a passenger in a car that needs to stop suddenly, and they become taut with a compulsion to escape when you are threatened. The flight impulse is felt keenly in the legs; it feels almost as if your very limbs were demanding that you run. They can tremble and feel wobbly under stress or become rigid with fear, a remnant of that animal tonic immobility that makes deer freeze in the road when cars approach them. On my recent drive to Montreal, undertaken with much trepidation, I had severe tension in my legs for the hour I drove through the region of flat farmland one encounters just over the border from Vermont. This is one of the many sequelae—accompanying symptoms—associated with anxiety. Part of one's task is to learn to accept such sensations and not compound them with additional fear. Since vast spaces affect me physically, I react to them even when I am just passing by them in a car.

I forget all these reactions when I am in secure surroundings. I feel myself to be "normal." I even pretend to myself—or is there truth in this?—that my "personality" (if one can distinguish such ingrained and self-defeating tendencies from "personality") is somehow incompatible with agoraphobia. Sometimes it feels like just an unfortunate fluke that I inherited this trait, as if a caramel sauce had been mistakenly poured over a leg of lamb by a cook who took it to be gravy. Agoraphobia *is* at odds with the tone of some of what I do. I am not wary in every domain. I teach at a college. I perform as a pianist. I can face a hostile audience playing a controversial piece of music or stand up to a group of colleagues at a faculty meeting and express a minority viewpoint. I write (or try to write) lively, expressive, outgoing music, and I can tolerate both good and bad reviews of my work.

Although I *have* improved in some ways over the years, the phobias are surprisingly intractable. At the same time I remember well the period before I experienced them and recall taking pleasure in some of the very things I now avoid. I have gradually reconstructed most of the situations in which I first experienced panic. One thing is clear: Simply discovering the experiential "origins" of the phobias does not free one from them, any more than discovering the reason why one resists practicing the piano would turn one suddenly into a better pianist. For that to occur, one would have to start practicing again. The same thing is true for phobias. The primary "cure" or help for them is in real-life practice, even if one *never* discovers when, where, and why they started.

What is perhaps most difficult to describe is how endangered one feels in the grip of such a reaction. The phobic response is inextricably blended with emotions and thoughts of death, separation, and loneliness. The chemical changes caused by the body's response to what it perceives as danger causes changes in the blood flow to, and the oxygen level of, the brain. The psychological and cognitive impact is real, and so is the aspect of reality—the precariousness of existence—that is stirred in the consciousness of the sufferer. I remember the strange, sad, and doom-laden expression on my father's face when our family car passed through a deserted mountainous area or an expanse of empty land, as if the shadow of death were passing over him. The outer vacuum

seemed to be seeping into his brain, as if he could not help inter-
nalizing the emptiness he saw outside the car window. He wore
the same expression when we passed the huge cemeteries that
lined the highway leading to what was then Idlewild (now JFK)
Airport, an expression that suggested that death was more immi-
nent when it was under discussion or in view. He was a serious
man, with a deep sympathy for human suffering and a capacity
for awe. But there was almost no boundary between his sensitivity to the mystery of life and his phobic terror of it. (In Hebrew,
incidentally, there is also no such differentiation; the same word is
used to connote both "awe" and "fear.")

The phobic's sense of boundaries is always porous. This is
why phobias and superstitions are akin. Both involve what some
psychiatrists call magical thinking. How does one differentiate
between the need to knock wood while giving thanks for being
healthy and the conviction that if one takes a local road, one will
be in a zone of safety, while on a highway there will be danger?
Or that if one carries a cell phone and a bottle of ginger ale, one
will be safer than without them?

The phobic not only becomes afraid of his own fearful
thoughts but also unconsciously believes that those very thoughts
will bring about changes in what happens. He believes, in a
quasi-superstitious way, that because he is afraid of the highway, it
is more likely that a traffic jam will occur while he is on it than
that it will occur when someone else is on it. (A very solipsistic
view of life!) At the same time the actual feelings and ideas stirred
by the phobic response are completely rational; they relate to the
very real terrors of being a human being. And since they connect
with the real, they make the places and circumstances that so
readily stimulate them seem truly dangerous. Because of the associative powers of the mind, the flavors of truth—the truth of our
mortality and of life's unpredictability—are folded into the dough

of anticipatory and interpretive fantasy. The daily bread of phobics is a strange mix of deep truth and magical thinking. It is true that we all will die and that, apparently alone among creatures, we know it. But it is not true that we are likely to die when on a highway or a bridge or in an elevator or in the subway or in any circumstance of which we have a phobia simply because we are in a state of panic about it. Those situations are not particularly dangerous, and neither is panic. Like a laugh track in a situation comedy, a custom-made, cognitive message of doom accompanies panic symptoms. But unlike a laugh track, the message can be talked down.

I spoke to an old friend, Fred, who is a psychologist. We have known each other since we were ten years old. I asked him what he made of my terror of being deep in the woods or of passing the silent, ancient surfaces of jagged rock lining roadways? What disaster was I fearing?

"We have certain sensitivities that allow us to learn an awful lot very quickly through what is called one-time learning," he told me. "Those then become templates for other overwhelming situations, and sometimes we misread later situations because we were overwhelmed at an earlier time."

He went on to talk about the implications of not being afraid, of, in the case of facing blankness, the desires unleashed in the blank space. "It's complicated," he said reflectively. "Take a fear of heights, for example. There are issues having to do with whether the person wants to stay in control. . . . There is not just the fear of falling but of the opposite impulse, to throw himself over.

"In considering your question, I find myself thinking about how many forces have both the positive and the negative in them. When you hold your hand up, there is the force pulling it down, but there are muscles when you are doing anything working in opposition to each other that make it steady. You need a pull in both directions to have accuracy and homeostasis of some sort, so that you always have this in various ways, both physical and psychologically. You keep your balance by also being willing to lose your balance. To take a step forward, you have to momentarily let go of your balance, as it were."

The philosopher Blaise Pascal, who has sometimes been described as an agoraphobic, wrote of the baffling haphazardness of being and of his fright facing the "eternal silence of infinite spaces": "When I consider the short duration of my life, swallowed up in the eternity before and after, the little space which I fill, and even can see, engulfed in the infinite immensity of spaces of which I am ignorant, and which know me not, I am frightened, and am astonished at being here rather than there; for there is no reason why here rather than there, why now rather than then. Who has put me here? By whose order and direction have this place and time been allotted to me?"

One can feel this silence looking up at the stars or at a vast expanse of ocean or even sitting alone in a room. At such moments one loses one's orientation. One listens for a reassuring sound and hears nothing. On the one hand, this is the most adult of feelings, being face-to-face with nothingness. On the other hand, it is something utterly primal, animal, and infantile, a sensation of abandonment, as if one were an infant left alone on a mountaintop to die.

Faced with an environment of wilderness, or what I perceive as emptiness, for any appreciable length of time, I begin to get my symptoms. The worst is probably the sensation of being unable to breathe properly (dyspnea). I react as if I cannot master my own breathing unless there are frequent signs of human life. I also feel my digestive system start to come unglued. At the same time my mind starts to "disintegrate," as if a magnet holding together the iron filings of coherent thought were suddenly removed and the filings dispersed. I have the impression of entering nonbeing itself.

In *The Concept of Anxiety* Søren Kierkegaard wrote about facing nothingness. He described anxiety as a kind of dizziness. To Kierkegaard, mankind is a psychical and physical being perched over an abyss. He can only achieve a synthesis of his two aspects by uniting in a third, in his spirit. Because he is free, he can resist looking down into the abyss, but "he who looks down into the yawning abyss becomes dizzy. But what is the reason for this? It is just as much in his own eye as in the abyss, for suppose he had not looked down. Hence anxiety is the dizziness of freedom, which emerges when the spirit wants to posit the synthesis and freedom looks down into its own possibility, laying hold of finiteness to support itself. Freedom succumbs in this dizziness."

In a sense, a phobia can be seen as a kind of fissure in reality, opened up by a reaction that is either out of sync with what stimulates it or, as with the fear of open spaces and heights, overly sympathetic to it.

On an ocean liner to England in 1990, my fourth and most recent trip to Europe as of this writing, I coped with the dread of the vastness by going to the ballroom dance classes and attending movies, lectures, and even an onboard piano recital. I can remember the sickening mixture a Chopin nocturne made in the pit of my stomach with the roiling of the featureless ocean outside, and write my eerie sensations of isolation and captivity. My busy schedule held the tiny iron filings of my psyche together like a magnet, but only barely. And to think that I was there because my fear of planes was still more severe than my fear of being on the ocean!

One night, as happens from time to time on a crossing, there was an extraordinary fog that obliterated the ocean entirely. Every two minutes a bass-voiced foghorn resonated from the ship's stem into the mysterious white mist, like a question. The moonlight fell on the dark curtain of fog, lighting it strangely. It was as if the ship were wrapped in a cocoon and lost in a void as deep below as above, as deep before as behind. I held panic at bay by focusing on the meticulously timed sounding of the primal foghorn as if it alone established a sense of coherence in the world.

In a ship on the ocean one is surrounded by human society and closer than usual to "help." There is all one needs of human experience inside, but outside there is night. This night reminds us: However full of inner resources we may be and however many outer connections we may have, we as individuals are still absolutely, irrevocably singular. Our brief life span is bounded on all sides by nothingness. The lively earth moves through the infinite dark.

I actually enjoy driving if I am on the routes that I know well. At times, driving through the hills and small towns in Vermont, I experience an almost erotic ecstasy, a feeling of escape and adventure. When I am listening to exciting music (such as Dutch composer Louis Andriessen's *De Stijl*), I sometimes inadvertently accelerate to match the tempo of the work. I have gotten my share of speeding tickets. I learned to drive right before the birth of my daughter; I thought that I had better know how to drive if I was going to be a father! I took lessons on the streets of New York with a wonderful man from the South, Mr. Woods, who wore green checked pants, the kind of man you would trust with your entire life savings while you went to do an errand. A grandfather himself, he was extremely amused by my excited anticipation of having a child, and he was an excellent, steady teacher. His advice has stuck with me, and I still hear his voice in my head when I make decisions at the wheel.

I am completely unfazed by driving in New York City traffic (now that *is* truly irrational). But not only will I not drive on highways, for the most part, but as the reader knows, if I am called upon to drive anywhere new, I am in the absurd position of having to rehearse the drive first to see if I can handle it. Many times I can't. Sometimes I have to try a ride many times before I get past a point where I am stuck, a stretch of steep mountain, say, bounded on all sides by layered slabs of rock (how long will it go on like this?), or the beginning of a bridge whose length I can't judge from the available view (it could be long or lead to a confusing mass of coiled ramps, and I might take the wrong one and be on a highway that has no exit for the next thirty miles).

Sometimes I keep a log on a yellow pad next to me on the drive to a new place, to help me cope with the experience. Jotting down my thoughts centers me, and noting everything I pass furnishes me with a kind of Ariadne's thread for the return trip. Even to me, back home at my computer, my reaction to the road seems in retrospect ludicrous, even laughable; the psychic pain I see demonstrated in the jottings on the pad makes me flinch. Like most people, I delight in mentally reliving the details of pleasure—a romantic encounter, a sunlit picnic—but jettison pain from the memory as soon as I am free of it. I don't want to admit that this is a part of who I am, and I would really prefer to forget all these sensations and thoughts once they are over. Many of my pad jottings are absurdly specific, about the drive itself and things seen through the car window, names of stores and signs scrawled in a shaky hand:

Quail Hollow Inn . . .
Yankee Pet Supply ("Got Pups? You Bet") . . .
Cold River Industrial Park . . .
Sign: "Corn" . . .
Chuck's Auto . . .

City Auto . . .
Tom and Dale's Auto . . .
Church (sign: " 'Everybody's doing it' doesn't make it right")
Noise "R" Us Fireworks . . .
Wendell Marsh . . .

When I see these same signs on the return trip, I am deeply reassured and also surprised that everything has stayed put. The fear creates a dreamlike state; it helps to see the concrete world corroborated. The place-specific notations seem to demonstrate an effort to maintain a sense of reality and a sense of identity while in transit, as if my identity and sense of control were at risk, as if I were, like a Star Trek character, being "beamed" from one location to another, with my molecular reconstruction at the new location less than certain. This must relate to the feeling of disintegration called depersonalization. Is this travel response actually part of all normal experience of travel but perceived by most people as only mild nervousness or as part of the excitement? Apparently my antennae for certain inner frequencies are on the wrong setting, so that what strikes other ears as the tinkling of a small bell has for me the impact of a deafening gong. Yet I also from time to time travel with only minimal anxiety, feeling like "myself" the entire time. What a revelation that is! Apparently travel does not have to be some kind of psychic high wire act.

The study of abnormality often sheds light on the workings of the normal. The locus of a brain injury in patients who have mental or physical deficits have revealed to neurologists where the brain centers for the normally functioning faculties are. I often think that phobias reveal something about the human need for familiarity, by representing a flawed or attenuated working of the faculty of habituation. The difference in my perceptions of the very same road between the first time I travel it, the return trip, and subsequent trips can be startling. Some roads always remain daunting or, regrettably, even "impassable." Safety seems to be connected with the notion of something "belonging" to me. It is as if with repeated journeys my consciousness gradually "marked" each passing landmark with its own presence, the way a dog marks trees with his urine. As I relax about the route, I notice more and more reasons to find it human and habitable. Eventually my vigilance subsides, and I cease to pay much attention to it at all. This seems like nothing but an exaggerated form of the kind of habituation with which we live our lives from day to day, moment to moment.

Nature clearly means for us to have the ability to adapt to the world and to find it "normal." Without this capacity we couldn't focus on our foreground activities. We couldn't survive if we did not have the ability to turn our attention to immediate necessities. This requires our taking our surroundings for granted unless they are threatening.

We could almost say that our sense of "security" and "safety" represents a reprieve from uneasiness, a form of denial, that when we are feeling safe, we are simply inured to the strangeness of life, so that we can function within it and cope with the things we need to cope with. By this definition, our equanimity could be seen as a kind of desensitization, and our phobias not so much as aberrant but as a resurgence of sensitivity at an inopportune time. When we encounter the unfamiliar—a creature with eight legs or an unaccustomed environment—we have thrust back in front of us our own strangeness. Such feelings can be aroused surprisingly easily—by horror films, for example. One particularly effective technique in such stories is to situate them in surroundings that are initially reassuring—a tranquil, "safe" community in which there are "typical" families etc. When within these settings, alien creatures appear, horrifying diseases are unleashed, and psychotic transformations occur, everyday life is gradually unmasked as potentially out of control and horrific. For the suggestible among us it can take an entire night of bad dreams to reinstate a sense of normality.

Children tend to be wary of anything new. They love repetition: the familiar song sung every night, again and again. Their brains are primed to be reassured by the structure of the human face—that is why they will smile even at a drawing of a circle, two eyes, and a mouth—but quickly differentiate between the faces they know and those they don't. "Stranger anxiety" is the very first phobia, and it strikes most children toward the end of their first year, at about the time they are becoming mobile enough to encounter many new faces. Even an unfamiliar vegetable on a dinner plate may elicit a protest from a small child.

Habituation makes it possible for us to place things and experiences in a relation to ourselves that is tolerable. It would appear that we have the desire to domesticate everything we see, which is to say identify ourselves with it in some way. The revulsion caused in some of us by snakes, for example, may in part be the result of our difficulty identifying ourselves with them. We connect with the snake as an animate being but shrink at reconciling our form with its form. Perhaps it is actually the identification that fuels the revulsion. At the same time the snake's historical dangerousness has left an imprint on our instincts. We are certainly less likely to recoil when we see a toy train set.

Our routines inure us to the strangeness of the world. Traveling exposes us to it once more. Even hearing of alien ideas and customs obliges us to see ourselves in a larger context that renders our own customs, our lives, our very selves more *arbitrary*. Our natural need to be comfortable with ourselves and our world is perpetually at odds with the reality that we might just as easily have been born here as there, this racial or national type as that one, in this country as that one, in this income bracket as that one, or even as a nonhuman animal.

As a child one has an almost visceral tendency to shrink from what is unfamiliar, as if from a threat. Whatever is slightly abnormal within a given perspective is scary because it shows an alternate possibility: *This can happen; this could be you.* This tendency asserts itself when children mock a child who is overweight or, like my sister, mentally deficient. I remember being at summer camp and seeing the retarded boys—there were, for some reason, always one or two retarded children there each summer—pushed around and jeered at by the bigger, supposedly savvier kids. In retrospect, it seems clear that this expressed fear along with the sadistic impulses, elicited by superior strength, that make children pull the wings off flies. There is a link between our unconscious discomfort with the oddness of our own natures and forms, our need for reinforcement of our own "normality," and many forms of intolerance. Seeing someone so like oneself, yet ever so slightly different, reveals the accident of one's own characteristics, places one back in nature. As with animal phobias, we squirm, in part, because we think, "I could just as well have been born a creature like that." Sometimes this squirming turns punitive.

After seeing the original movie version of *The Fly,* as well as after seeing a horror movie about rats, I had trouble shaking off the unpleasant feeling that I might in fact be turning into one of those creatures. As I drifted off to sleep, I wondered if the arm under my pillow had not become the hairy limb of an insect and worried that if I looked too quickly in the bathroom mirror, I might see a rodent's beady eyes looking back.

Bigotry has always made much use of animal comparisons in its stereotyping of despised groups. It is the "other" that is an "animal." It is the "other" type of sexuality that is "disgusting." Among other things, bigotry seems to express a displaced self-loathing. Prejudice surely shares some features with phobia, though in two respects it is distinct: It is characterized primarily by aggression, and no one seeks treatment for it.

Like phobias, racism, homophobia, sexism, and xenophobia would appear to be the channeling of deep anxieties and fears into inappropriate objects. When Europeans blamed the Gypsies or Jews for their troubles, or Americans identified this or that immigrant population as a danger to the American way of life, this could be interpreted as a way they gave their inchoate fears a "manageable" shape. Like phobias, such fantasies are often the result of, or maintained by, negative conditioning in the form of propaganda and myths. At the same time, unlike phobias, they arouse much more of a fight than a flight response. At their most severe they constitute a pathology leading to rage and persecution. At the heart of such oppression lies a fear.

One could make the case that sexism on the part of males constitutes a thinly veiled fear of self, a terror not of difference but of *sameness*, which stimulates an urgent need to distinguish oneself from an "other." In the case of homophobia, perhaps fear is also a kind of distancing mechanism. It would certainly seem that fear of male homosexuality is most pronounced in men.

If treatment was sought for ethnic and gender biases, it would probably take the same form as treatment for phobias. Those who are schooled in diverse communities, or who have served as soldiers or athletes alongside unfamiliar groups eventually learn the limits and absurdities of stereotyping.

While driving, I am comforted by seeing houses by the side of the road—"homes," as it were. In German the word *heimlich* means "not strange, familiar, tame, dear." In his essay "The Uncanny" Freud reminded us that the German word *unheimlich* ("uncanny") literally means "unhomelike." "One would suppose, then, that the uncanny would always be an area in which a person was unsure of his way around," he writes. "The better oriented he was in the world around him, the less likely he would be to find the objects and occurrences in it uncanny." But Freud went on to show that in fact the word *heimlich* can under certain conditions be used to mean that which "was intended to remain secret, hidden away . . . inscrutable." The word *heimlich* can sometimes acquire "the sense that otherwise belongs to 'unheimlich.'" In a brilliant line of reasoning he added that the sensation of the uncanny particularly applies to deeply rooted, buried, *familiar* things, things "long familiar to the psyche" but "estranged" from it by being repressed. In this category belongs the fear of the dead and of ghosts. As modern people we have only theoretically surmounted our belief in spirits. In fact, wrote Freud, our emotional reactions to death have changed little since primitive times. After all, science has remained unable to describe the firsthand experience of dying or even to disabuse us of our instinctive intimations of a possible afterlife. Our unconscious is "still as unreceptive as ever to the idea of our own mortality." In the dark, in silence, at the hint of unexplained sounds in a graveyard, our latent uncertainty about the nature of death reemerges.

It is precisely this kind of uncertainty about what is possible in the real world, or the revelation of unsuspected properties in the *familiar*, stated Freud, which initiates the sense of uncanniness.

Freud mentioned in particular the uncanny effect of epilepsy and madness, "a manifestation of forces that [the layman] did not suspect in a fellow human being, but whose stirrings he can dimly perceive in remote corners of his own personality." At such moments our perception of the possible is shaken, and "the boundary between reality and fantasy is blurred."

Traveling can elicit such feelings, stirring primal fears of the enormous, exciting, arbitrary, diverse natural world that we in fact do live in, but of which we generally view only a small piece. Perhaps these fears lie dormant in us, like streptococcus bacteria, ready to be aroused by what is unfamiliar. How can it be—we ask ourselves—that for some people *this* alien place is home, *this* their daily view—one so familiar that they no longer even look at it—*this* their idea of "normality"? Many of my notes to myself in my makeshift traveling log suggest a preoccupation with the mystery of being in another context:

reassuring tethers to and confirmations of external reality: "Subaru"; "Delio Sports"; "PetCo" . . .

feeling a member of society dwindles so easily

connections to self, past, others . . . vanish in the forest

places you pass on the road gradually become personalized . . .

there's an emotional quality to interpreting the landscape—on the way (nervous) I thought: "This house looks abandoned" on the way back (more relaxed) I thought: "People are probably home. Maybe they are making dinner" . . .

when I start to relax, let down my guard, then the terror hits

how can I observe this tree, this path, this house— only now, at this moment—yet it has been there for a century?

Once the context has been made familiar by many return trips, the same road I initially traveled with such apprehension and caution becomes almost invisible, simply a backdrop for getting from here to there, a nonissue. All the dark images and memories turn into a thin cloud of smoke easily whisked back into the genie's bottle of the imagination. I observe this lightening of my load with amazement.

The cognitive behavioral therapists made a momentous discovery in the 1980s, when they found that many people with agoraphobia and many specific phobias have a fear of the physical and psychological effects of fear which is stronger than their dread of the context in which they experience them. It meant that the task of cure can in some cases be simplified into demystifying fear, and learning not to aggravate its symptoms. After many years of being told so, I have finally begun to understand that the tangled thoughts accompanying my irrational fears are merely the sparks thrown off by the grinding machinery of panic when it has no external cause. Beneath all the philosophizing on my notepad, beneath the "ideational content" (as the psychologists put it) of my anxious searching and catastrophizing, is actually the anxiety of being far from help when the panic itself hits. When one can remove the sting of the panic—through therapy, practice, medication, or simple understanding—one can actually face the phobic trigger without that sense of doom, even when the dread has become so ingrained

as to have begun to seem virtually rational. One discovers that being "near help" is not necessary after all, that one isn't so far from
"home" after all, that one's surroundings are not after all "un-
homey," since one carries safety in oneself. But then one also has to
be prepared to dismantle all that has grown up around these fears
and to face their personal significance and usefulness.

Chapter Eight

Conditioning

Or as, when an underground train, in the tube, stops too
long between stations,
And the conversation rises and slowly fades into silence
And you see behind every face the mental emptiness deepen
Leaving only the growing terror of nothing to think about. . . .

I said to my soul, be still, and wait without hope
For hope would be hope for the wrong thing. . . .
—T. S. ELIOT, "EAST COKER"

The capacity to experience anxiety and the capacity to plan
are two sides of the same coin.
—DAVID BARLOW

For the past few years I have lived with a cat, Kiwi, in the house.
I have become increasingly aware of the range of her communicating behaviors, ability to learn, and capacity to size up new situations. I can see her tremendous skill at coping with her
environment and sense her emotional sensitivity. Yet I am also
aware that in many ways her cognitive and affective life differs
dramatically from mine. Her learning and thinking abilities are,
it would appear, matched to the life she leads. She has memorized the smells and shapes of every corner of the house and
every pathway to it, is able to return faithfully—sometimes hag-

gard, disheveled, and covered with shredded shards of leaves—from a day's distant exploring and hunting. Her ears straighten with attention at noises far beneath my threshold of perception. At the murmur of a car engine half a mile away she readies herself to get out of the road and out of harm's way. She darts with lightning speed at a moving insect form no wider than a thread. Intuiting the presence of another cat in the field outside, she leaps with curiosity onto the windowpane. She hides under a chair with discouragement when she sees me packing my suitcase in preparation for time away from her. She stays completely still while I am playing a piece on the piano and intrudes only after the last note has died away. She has an uncanny sense of balance and a natural ability to right herself when she lands on her padded paws after falling from a height. She instinctively pats down the litter in the litter box before urinating and then covers the urine over afterward so that neither prey nor predator who might come upon it sees that she is nearby.

Kiwi is a student of what pertains to her. She has learned how my voice sounds when directed at her from far away and knows that the sound of the can opener opening a tin, or of a fork on a plate, might mean that she is about to be fed. Naturally, she can't know from the sound if the can is truly meant for her, but at the first inkling of the metallic timbre she comes into the kitchen to check. I assume that she also experiences an excited sense of anticipation and the physiological preparations for eating at the noise.

At the turn of the twentieth century the Russian neurophysiologist I. P. Pavlov began his now-famous studies of reflex responses in animals, researches that eventually culminated in a series of celebrated lectures he gave in 1924 in Petrograd (St. Petersburg). Studying the "unconditioned" salivation mechanism in dogs when they were fed, one of the innate (unconditioned) reflexes human and nonhuman animals are born with, he realized that the dogs salivated not only while eating but also when the food was placed at some distance away and was accessible only to sight and smell. They salivated when they saw the plate that normally contained the food, when they saw the person who normally brought the plate, and when they heard the footsteps of the person who normally fed them. (This anticipatory salivation is beneficial in that it prepares animals to digest the food or, in the event that what they taste is poisonous or noxious, to spit it out easily.)

Pavlov experimented with the ringing of a bell each time he was about to feed the dogs, and after the dogs had become accustomed to the connection between the sound of the bell and the appearance of food, they salivated whenever they heard the bell whether or not they were fed. He called this a conditioned reflex. Conditioned reflexes are those that we acquire from experience, and they are at the root of all our learned associations and responses. By this means we still instinctively "train" or teach animals to come when we call them or answer commands.

Thus Pavlov demonstrated that a conditioned reflex, such as the response to the sound of the bell, could easily be superimposed upon an unconditioned reflex, the natural salivation in response to food. He then showed that a conditioned reflex could also be revised or unlearned—i.e., a buzzer could replace the bell. Most important in terms of our subject, he demonstrated that a conditioned *negative* reflex could be created by subjecting an animal to an unwanted stimulus when it performed a specific activity; an animal would avoid going where it had received a shock or heard a loud noise.

Conditioning actually mimics the way the brain teaches us to remember what is dangerous. When we touch a flame, our motor reflexes act instantaneously to remove our hand and only later send the message to the brain that we have been hurt. It is the brain's pain signal that makes us remember not to touch the flame in the future. Injury itself is distinct from the sensation of pain. A paralyzed person, placed in a hot bathtub, can watch his skin burning without feeling sensations. Pain is our internal conditioning shock, teaching us what to avoid.

In this very way a person can quickly learn to associate his own anxiety sensations to the situations in which he has felt them—to respond to his painful symptoms during a subway ride or a drive over a bridge or when he sees a spider, as if the symptoms were electric shocks or buzzers teaching him to avoid these things. Such "learning" becomes all the more powerful when fueled by traumatic circumstances, since it then becomes burned into the most instinctive part of the brain. But even events experienced vicariously (a subway accident heard of on the evening news, the sight of a friend fleeing in terror from a spider) can reinforce our dreads in a primitive way.

Although some of Pavlov's terminology is out of date, his basic conclusions about how we learn what to approach and what to avoid from our first days on earth hold true. We are formed by what we learn. We discover not only what will bring about the satisfaction of our needs, but what some of those needs are. Our lives are a narrative made up of millions of learning experiences, which either confirm us in our likes and dislikes or retrain us in them.

When we speak of bonding between parent and child, between teacher and student, between patient and doctor, or between friends, perhaps we are really speaking of something that begins as a kind of conditioned response, a positive feeling to which we want to return. As a parent one hopes that sooner or later the child will connect with something and bond with an interest: sports, science, music—i.e., discover that an area of interest satisfies inner needs and aptitudes that are, as it were, revealed in the child's encounters with it. When I heard Stravinsky's *Le Sacre du Printemps,* Schoenberg's "Six Little Pieces," and Bartok's Sixth String Quartet for the first time, the music resonated with my genetic makeup and with many things already implanted in me by my upbringing. The next time I had the opportunity to listen to music, I was attracted, excited, and joyful. It makes sense to think of this as a kind of positive conditioning, an association between a positive emotion and an activity, which stimulates further involvement with the activity, which in turn reinforces the initial bond.

If we stop to think about it, we even bond with our most trivial possessions, some of which over time become tied to us through such a complex network of associations and memories that they seem almost to possess souls. The sentimental value we attach to our red stuffed elephant Pete reinforces our sense of our own past, our own reality, our own value.

Michelle, the student of developmental psychology, put it to me this way: "Genetics directs the formation of all of these neurons and where they are going to wind up, that there will be a connection of neurons that elicit movement, neurons that are in your spinal cord that are going to come up into your brain, neurons that are going to elicit a more conscious response to things, neurons that are providing sensory information, and so forth. You have all of these different types of neurons, designed genetically so that they will all connect in a certain way, and the specific maps are pretty similar from person to person. Yet we are all modulated by our experiences."

There is powerful evidence that some phobias are acquired easily while others depend upon more specific conditioning, modeling, or personal associations. In other words, just as we are predisposed to gravitate *toward* nourishment or sexual partners, so our brains may be prewired to quickly learn to flee certain potential threats. A celebrated series of experiments conducted on monkeys by Susan Mineka at the University of Wisconsin showed that a negative reaction to snakes could be instilled in innocent laboratory-raised monkeys simply by showing them films of older monkeys in the wild reacting in terror to snakes. However, the same laboratory monkeys, shown a film that through editing made their role models appear to cringe at the sight of flowers, did not imitate this response. An experiment conducted on an infant boy, Little Albert, by the early-twentieth-century behaviorist J. B. Watson, in which the appearance of a white rat was accompanied by a loud metal noise, left the infant in one stroke afraid of "rats, dogs and anything furry, even fur coats." (Also, no doubt, afraid of Dr. Watson.) But in experiments conducted in later times, the loud metallic noise did not instill a dread of such objects as curtains, blocks, or wooden ducks.

Some proponents of an evolutionary theory of fear, like the Swedish researcher Arne Öhman, have even tried to demonstrate that ancient fears, such as a fear of the dark or of snakes, stir deeper responses in the reptilian brain and are therefore more intractable than those more recent in origin, such as the fear of guns. Martin Seligman of the University of Pennsylvania found that birds are "prepared" to fear cats and not people, despite the fact that in modern times people are an equal threat to them. Although still other experimenters have disputed the distinction between ancient and modern fears, most of us would probably relate instinctively to the notion that certain fears are "primal." What is indisputable is that we are primed for fear itself and subject to the influence of both experience and example (i.e., the fear reactions of our parents) in the development of our fear responses. If our mother always screamed, "Be careful!"

when we saw dogs, we are surely more likely to respond in Little Albert fashion and to have developed a wariness near them. It also turns out that negative associations can be formed much more easily than positive ones, and for very good reason. For survival, learning what is harmful needs to be easy. At the same time, according to some theorists, animals are "contraprepared" to make the association between an instinctive activity, like the pecking done by birds, and a bad result. That is to say that whereas pigeons can easily learn to peck on a key to receive food, they can't learn to disassociate the activity of pecking from feeding, even when experiments are designed to teach them that pecking a key causes their food *not* to appear. They can learn what to avoid as harmful but can't be taught that their pecking instinct is counterproductive.

Post-Pavlovian experiments have confirmed that animals can be conditioned to avoid an object or place—anything, in fact—if it becomes associated with something painful (a small electric shock, a loud noise, an unpleasant taste) and that they can be very gradually *re*conditioned to approach the same object or place if it is slowly reintroduced, step by step, in an attractive context (associated with desirable food, etc.). They need to be motivated to reapproach it, but when they do, are rewarded, and suffer no deleterious effects, their confidence about its safety can be restored.

It makes sense that the normal human alarm system would be a bit oversensitive. But studies suggest that people with anxiety disorders dispel their fear reactions much more slowly than the nonanxious, even when it is demonstrated to them that their fears have been artificially stimulated by the studies themselves.

Fear is contagious, particularly when modeled by a parent, but it can also be communicated in films and literature. Cultural norms as well play their role in shaping our imaginations, helping determine whether we squirm at the sight of spiders, as many Americans and Japanese do; eat them as delicacies, as Australian aborigines do; or keep them as pets, as some children in Brazil do.

It is remarkable how easily a sensation of creepiness can be communicated. (Note that the word "creepy" derives from the crawling of insects and snakes.) The mechanisms of associative fear can be felt at work around a campfire, where the darkness and isolation of the setting can be played upon by a scary story as if they were the strings of a lyre, made to sound a music of dread. In a horror movie, visual, musical, and associative techniques can unnerve our sensibilities in a few seconds. Alfred Hitchcock's masterful film *The Birds* almost succeeds in instilling ornithophobia in the audience.

Our imaginations are clearly malleable, and the distinction between reality and fantasy is, in a sense, a secondary process to response. Mind and body begin to react whether or not an event, object, or idea is actually present. Without this receptivity, dreams, ritual, and art would not exist. These days brain imaging can allow neurologists to watch the brain in action. Experiments have shown that we recognize angry faces more quickly than neutral ones—presumably the quicker to fight, submit, or get out of the way. Amazingly, in experiments that examined the neural activity in the amygdalas of subjects who were shown pictures of angry and neutral faces, there was a clear response in the brain to the angry faces even when they were shown too quickly to be consciously perceived. In other words, the "mind" was preparing for an appropriate response to anger *even before* the subjects were aware of the stimulus. Propaganda has long made use of our ability to be molded by powerful imagery, both positive and negative. Americans have made propaganda targets of Native Americans, Germans, Japanese, and many other groups.

The German propaganda machine in the Nazi era was able to cultivate a distaste for the Jews, making use of the public's latent germ phobia (and hundreds of years of anti-Semitic prejudice and lore) to demonize Jews as a contaminant of "Aryan" blood.

Filmmaker François Truffaut used the futuristic Ray Bradbury novel *Farenheit 451* to convey a message about fascism, propaganda, and mass hysteria. In the film the actor Oscar Werner portrays a "fireman" whose job is to burn the books being secretly hoarded by a literate underground in a society where books are forbidden. The allusion to the book burnings in Nazi Germany is underscored by the casting of the German Werner in the role. The movie shows with great subtlety how virtually anything, including a book, can become the object of fear if it is surrounded by the behaviors associated with dread.

As the author Annette Insdorf points out, Truffaut subliminally conveyed the idea that written language is taboo in the film's very first frames, which plung us into an aliterate world in which even the title and credits intended for us, the viewers, are narrated rather than printed. We see printed words for the first time only in the scene when firemen emerge from a house carrying large net bags containing books to be confiscated and destroyed. In the piles of illicit material, the titles *Don Quixote* and *Memoirs of Charlie Chaplin* and the name Oscar Wilde are fleetingly visible. Families from antiseptically identical houses emerge to gaze with appalled fascination at the stack of books from a distance. At one point, in a scene of searching for contraband books, a woman knocks against a picture frame and leaps away when a book falls from behind it, as frightened as Tippi Hedren is by the bird that appears suddenly from behind a picture frame in a parallel moment of Hitchcock's *The Birds.*

Advertisers try to instill in us chains of positive associations, relying on our tendency to salivate when we see a picture of a hamburger and trying to extend our associations from the hamburger to the logo of the restaurant selling it to more primal satisfactions—sex, affluence, happiness, security, comradeship. Their goal is that we, like Pavlov's dogs salivating at the bell, will feel longing when we see the logo all by itself.

The millions of small connections we make between the objects and activities in the world and our memories, ideas, and emotions about them come close to constituting our sense of self. We happily note the effects of a whiff of perfume or a familiar tune in reanimating whole constellations of poignant or pleasant images from our past, but such sense memories and processes of association can just as easily be distressing. The phobic response that reactivates an earlier discomfort feels almost like an uncoupling from this sense of self, as we instinctively back away from our mental processes, focusing only on the object of our fear.

Freud recognized that phobias can sometimes be instilled by a single shock. This may be even more likely when a jolting experience rekindles an already latent sense of danger. An instance of this is recounted in the story of a woman who went diving in a lake and swam directly into a corpse lying in the sludge at the water's bottom. This sudden fright understandably caused her subsequent avoidance of water. One can almost picture the instantaneous neurological fusion that must have occurred in her brain between the horror she encountered, the setting, the panic she felt, and the activity in which she was involved at the time she encountered it. This alone might surely be enough to create a phobic reaction in anyone, regardless of her predispositions. Only a deliberate relearning of the unlikelihood of the occurrence, a studied uncoupling of the negative associations between its elements, would cure her. How quickly she could accomplish this would depend upon all of the many variables in her makeup.

A young friend told me recently that he had become claustrophobic, like his father, after experiencing the terror of being held hostage in a bank holdup in his hometown. Perhaps in his case the trauma awakened a tendency to phobia that otherwise would have remained dormant.

At their most extreme, shocking experiences result in posttraumatic stress syndrome. But shocks need not be experienced firsthand to leave anxiety or phobias in their wake. The loss of his friend Henriette "Jette" Wulff in a conflagration on the transatlantic ship *Austria* left Hans Christian Andersen with a morbid fear of fire, a fear he captured in several stories, including "The Tin Soldier." Wullf's death affected him all the more because he learned that she had suffocated in her cabin, struggling to get out. Andersen, who suffered from a number of phobias and obsessions, already had a horror of being buried alive. In fact he kept, in all seriousness, next to his bedside a note that read "I only appear to be dead," lest he be mistaken for a corpse. In the wake of Wulff's violent end, he found it difficult to expunge from his mind the image of her small, struggling form (she was, incidentally, hunchbacked) and thereafter always carried a rope with him, to escape in the event of a fire.

One can imagine that the televised images of the collapse of the World Trade Center and its victims jumping to their deaths left a traumatic impact on many who saw them from far away, particularly children. It would be no exaggeration to say that the dropping of atomic bombs on Hiroshima and Nagasaki altered forever those who participated in the events on either side and that by changing our perception of the possible left a psychic scar on the entire human race. Such horrors leave psychological repercussions even on distant witnesses, inspiring "displaced" fears. Akira Kurosawa's film *Rhapsody in August* illustrates the effects of such a shock on a fictional character, a grandmother who still lives on the outskirts of central Nagasaki a few miles from the school where, forty-five years earlier, her husband died in the blast of the atom bomb. In one scene she recalls to her grandchildren how she ran outside when the sky was lit up by what seemed a colossal bolt of lightning, only to watch a gigantic mushroom cloud rising over the city. Now, in 1990, in the days following a commemoration of the destruction, the trauma returns to her. In confusion, she reacts in terror to a nighttime thunderstorm, which has merged in her mind with the horror that fell from the sky on August 9, 1945. She frantically tries to cover her grandchildren with a white sheet as they sleep and in a state of panic runs outside into the pouring rain.

In terms of confronting the normal hazards of life, there is certainly much wisdom in the old advice to get right back on the horse that threw you. An experience that swiftly contradicts a trauma can help the brain heal itself that much more quickly. Recent studies seem to suggest that the taking of antianxiety medication within the first hours after a traumatic episode helps stave off posttraumatic stress syndrome. It appears that the intervention of a physically relaxed state close to the experience alters the neurological connections that form around it.

Not every negative experience should lead to future avoidance. Our complex lives are full of suffering, and it requires subtle judgment to determine what each painful experience should teach us. If we burn ourselves touching the stove, that might mean that stoves should never be touched, or it might only mean that they shouldn't be touched under certain circumstances. If all we possessed was a mechanism for not repeating what hurts, we would never touch the stove again. We also need to be able to judge when pain is simply worth it, despite its inevitability, as in childbirth, a risky rescue attempt, or an act of defiance against authority.

Conditioning all by itself can't possibly explain the array of bizarre phobias we experience and can't explain why some people are riddled with phobias and others are free of them. Conditioning is a poor explanation of fears acquired without precipitating experiences or modeling. In so many cases, we discover a phobia in our very first encounters with an experience or, seemingly out of the blue, after many previously benign encounters. And conditioning doesn't help us understand why many who have had nasty experiences—being bitten by a dog, for example—*do not* subsequently develop phobias.

However, the concept of conditioning does at least partially account for the difficulty we often have overcoming the dread we feel once we have a phobia, since to learn fear is manifestly easier than to unlearn it. Nature has apparently arranged for us to be a little more on our guard than we might need to be since recklessness is more dangerous than apprehension.

Like Kiwi, each of us started life with a brain constrained both by the evolution of our species and by our individual genetic makeup. This brain has then been taught by life, its very pathways formed and strengthened by use, weakened by disuse. Through living, millions of cross-related associations, most of them forever hidden from conscious perception, all of them with physical ramifications, have accrued in the brain to the things and experiences of the world, leaving what feel like auras. When I sit down to the piano to compose, I am with the counterpoint assignments I handed in too late to my college theory professor; with the pieces once brought to joyous fruition and with those I abandoned or completed badly; I am with my father, my mother, my sister, my brother tuning his violin, my piano teacher on a Saturday at home in her Chinese dressing gown; with the Mozart concerto I learned at sixteen, with the Berg Piano Sonata, with the Fugue in C Sharp Minor of J. S. Bach. When I am on a train heading into a tunnel, I am engulfed by images of death and darkness, as if pinned beneath a gigantic calamitous wave. From moment to moment we relive our learning and build upon it.

Chapter Nine

Tigers in the Mind

Nothing so fixes a thing so intensely in the memory as the wish to
forget it.
—MICHEL DE MONTAIGNE

Not long ago, looking with identification and admiration at a
reproduction of Edvard Munch's 1893 painting *The Scream*, I
found myself wondering what Sigmund Freud would have had
to say about the painting and about Munch himself. The two
men were born a mere six years apart, Freud in 1856, Munch in
1863. Freud, the master of psychological excavation, was also
a collector of ancient Egyptian and Greek artifacts, and an astute
observer of painting, who wrote penetrating works about
Leonardo da Vinci and Michelangelo. It isn't difficult to imagine
Munch seeking out Freud's help. What would Freud have had to
say about the relationship between the painter's psychological
torments, his art, and the formative life events that marked him?

A series of family deaths apparently left deep imprints on
Munch's psyche, beginning with the death of his mother, when

he was five, the death of his favorite sister, Sophie, when he was fifteen (both from tuberculosis), and the loss of his father, an obsessive, devout, and moralistic physician, in 1889, when the painter was a rebellious young man. Following his father's death Munch entered a period of intense melancholy and emotional instability. Traveling alone in France, he suffered from agoraphobia, in the narrow sense of the term, finding it difficult to cross a street, dreading open spaces, and feeling "great dizziness at the slightest height." During this time he created a series of allegorical drawings in which a solitary elderly figure is seen walking away from the viewer down a road in vanishing perspective. These illustrations seemed to combine the symbolic representation of death and loneliness with a sense of space and perspective that conveyed anxiety and vertigo. He eventually expressed this *platzschwindel* in a number of works, culminating in *The Scream*, perhaps the most well-known visual representation of anxiety in all of art, a painting whose imagery exists in studies, a lithograph, the 1893 painting, and several other versions. From 1899 to around 1909 he spent time in a sanatorium and underwent various forms of treatment. His little known last paintings leave the roiling turbulence of *The Scream* and its disturbing sunset behind, as if reaching for an elusive sense of stability. Two of his final works, *The Sun* and *Towards the Light*, are ecstatic visions of sunrise.

As is well known, *The Scream* originated in a personal experience of mystical intensity that Munch noted in his diary in 1892 and told friends he was determined to paint. He had been walking along a bridge with two friends when the sky seemed to become a "bloody red" from the setting sun. Exhausted, he leaned over the railing. "My friends walked on" he wrote. "I stood there, trembling with fright. And I felt a loud, unending scream piercing nature."

The structure of *The Scream*, which so powerfully communicates a state of existential ill-being, emerged in stages. In *Despair*, from 1892, a hunched, brooding, and featureless man looks over a bridge in the lower frame of the canvas, while two others walk away from him in the direction of a disturbing sky. One could also compare the sense of self-loss conveyed in *The Scream* with the merging of the faces in *The Kiss* painted that same year. In this work the lovers become a merged abstraction that, in the words of playwright Stanislaw Przybyszewski, looks "like a giant ear."

In *The Scream*, the central figure no longer stands and broods and looks down, as in *Despair*, but directly faces the viewer and engages him in his fright. His face is emblematic, skull-like, almost genderless. With his hands to his ears he exhibits a classic Darwinian "gesture of sudden fright," and his curved and distorted body echoes the swirling whorls of the doom-laden sky. In contrast to these waving, bending shapes, the severity of the straight lines depicting the wooden bridge, and the upright, stick-like figures of the distant friends, all seen as if from above, create a vertiginous effect.

The Scream could represent two sides of the mind. On the one hand the man conveys an infinity of terror. But not far from him are those who regard the very same scene with equanimity.

Perhaps this is a part of what makes the image so harrowing. The calmness of the others on the bridge indicates that the man is not actually screaming. He expresses the scream with his open mouth and bulging eyes, and he covers his ears as if to muffle the sound of his own cry. But the scream is not heard. It is not expressed by the wraithlike man in the foreground of the painting, but flows through him and is projected onto nature itself. In this way *The Scream* could serve as a representation not only of panic but of Freud's concept of displacement. The agony the man feels, lacking expression, becomes enlarged and projected onto the world around him.

It was Freud who first tried to scientifically study the workings of our inner lives of associations and memories, and who first attempted to find methods of helping people unlearn the patterns of behavior and feeling that were harming them. In a book that deals with universal as well as personal experiences, the reader might expect me to take a position on whether my life experiences, as opposed to the constitution I was born with, "caused" my current psychological problems. I am not qualified to answer the question, nor am I certain how one draws the line between the innate self and one's experiences. Of course I "feel" as if my personality traits result from my life experience. But whatever happened *to* me happened *in dialogue* with me. Surely my constitution, my body, gave out signals from the first moment daylight struck it how it wished to be treated, what it liked and disliked, tolerated and rejected. My layman's belief is therefore a cautious one: that had I been mistakenly switched with Karlheinz Stockhausen Junior in the hospital nursery, say, and been raised in a different family, and had entirely different formative experiences, my psychological problems would have taken a different form than they have but would have expressed the same inner weaknesses and sensitivities.

By training as a physician and neurologist, Freud only gradually developed his theory of mind out of the painstakingly close study of patients suffering from incapacitating physical ailments and mental states. He did not originally intend to make a distinction between mind and body. He considered that he was laying the groundwork for what scholar Frank J. Sulloway calls a biology of mind. He continually revised his theories right up until the end of his life in 1939, when suffering from cancer, he fled from the Nazis with his extended family to "die in freedom," as he put it, in London. He was well aware that techniques did not yet exist to confirm fully many of his observations from a physiological point of view and that the language he employed was at times, of necessity, schematic.

Freud developed his concept of psychoanalysis, a term he invented, during a period when modern techniques of brain imaging were almost a century away. The discovery of neurons and synapses occurred during the same time, the 1890s, in which he was at work on his early "Project for a Scientific Psychology," in which he tried to outline the mechanical, physical, neurological, and biological laws behind psychological phenomena. He did not consider this early work complete, and it was not included as part of his "complete works," in the original twenty-four-volume standard edition collected and edited by James Strachey. Freud thought that he was describing the principles of mental life occurring within the human organism. He considered psychology an extension of biology.

Freud's early work was in biological research, and his first published paper was on the neuroanatomy of an early form of fish, the ammocoetes *Petromyzon*. From the beginning he was fascinated by the nervous system, the interaction between our brains and the rest of us. When he first entered the practice of medicine, he published numerous papers on the human nervous system and became a leading authority on the subject of child cerebral paralysis. He settled definitively on a career in neurology when he was in his late twenties, but only after acquiring three years of clinical experience in the Vienna General Hospital, working in the departments of surgery, internal medicine, psychiatry, nervous diseases, dermatology, and ophthalmology. Quite early he developed a legendary reputation as a neuropathologist whose "detailed knowledge of the nervous system's structure and function" made him capable of locating with astonishing accuracy the location of lesions that caused symptoms.

Ten years before he began his formulation of psychoanalytic theory Freud studied with renowned French neurologist Jean-Martin Charcot, who employed hypnosis to explore the causes of such mental illnesses as split personality and such nervous disorders as hysteria. Charcot's work helped reveal that consciousness was multilayered. Hypnosis pointed to the existence of compartmentalized levels of consciousness as in sleeping and waking that could communicate with each other while remaining separate. (The word "hypnosis" derives from the name Hypnos, the Greek god of sleep.)

Before Charcot, hysterical patients suffering from such debilitating symptoms as seizures and paralysis that could not be physiologically explained were regarded either as hypochondriacs or as malingerers. Charcot demonstrated that these devastating symptoms were "real," but not organic in origin. Since they could be artificially engendered under hypnosis—by the suggestion of the hypnotist—they might also be caused by unconscious psychological means—through the unconscious will of the patient (autosuggestion). Freud later confirmed the validity of this idea by showing how, in many cases, hysterical paralysis often took a form that was actually anatomically implausible and did not follow the laws of neuroanatomy exhibited in organic cerebral paralysis. These and many other discoveries of the time paved the way for the formulation of psychology as a quasi-independent branch of neurology. Through the systematic study of behavior, Charcot, Freud, and others began to analyze the layered, multifaceted, and often hidden territory of mental life.

Freud's background in zoology, anatomy, and physiology prepared him to extend Darwin's *The Expressions of the Emotions in Man and Animals* into the realm of individual human experience and behavior. Positing that nothing people do or feel can be arbitrary, his writings explore how our smallest unintended gestures and personal expressions have complex specific meanings and are as significant as, or often much more significant than, anything we intend to express. His debt to Darwin was explicit. "Every affect . . . is only a reminiscence of an event," he commented to a colleague.

Freud's writings teem with examples of behavior from daily life, which he examines for their underlying psychological purpose. Just as dreams are expressions from within us, said Freud, so our smallest gestures, habits, and words tell the story of what is happening inside us if only we can decipher them. When we trip up in our speech and say "kill" instead of "fill," or when we grow inexplicably uncomfortable when a certain topic comes up in a conversation, or when we dream we are swallowed by a fish, we are expressing aspects of ourselves of which we are unaware and that have meaning within the context of what has happened to us. Freud developed, in effect, a kind of chaos theory for what had seemed the bewildering arbitrariness of human behavior and thought processes, positing an order and laws at work behind our intentions, our mistakes, our jokes and games, our transgressions, our actions, thoughts, moods, and fantasies.

Like Darwin, Freud saw no discontinuity between man and all life. Thus man's impulses, according to Freud, are of a piece with those of other creatures, no matter how he covers, disguises, or sublimates them or however much he represses his knowledge of this continuity. Just as our expressions are remnants of actions, so the forms appetites and urges take in man are remnants of their earlier evolutionary forms. Freud considered that what he uncovered in the "psyche" constituted a kind of "third blow" to the "narcissism" of man. The first came when Copernicus demonstrated that planet Earth was not the center of the universe. The second was caused by Darwin's demonstration that man was descended from earlier primates and, like them, the product of evolution. And the third was that we humans are not even masters of our own primitive drives. Just as there is no decisive break between humanity and the animal kingdom, so there is no clean break between a "good" person and an "evil" one; we all contain the potential for good and evil thoughts and actions. There is equally no solid break between those suffering from what we call mental illness and those who do not. Freud showed that even what we now call sexual preference is a matter of degree, deriving from the dominance of one side of our nature over the other.

Freud kept refining his thinking about anxiety and anxiety neuroses such as phobias and obsessive-compulsive disorder throughout his life. In trying to understand the reasons some people are more subject to anxiety and neurosis than others, he posited the same contributing factors that anxiety authority David Barlow and others investigate today, "a biological, a phylogenetic and a purely psychological factor"—in other words, one's individual biological endowments, the evolution of the species itself, and the contribution of personal history, beginning at, or even before, birth. His 1926 work *Inhibitions, Symptoms, and Anxiety* includes both a discussion of Alfred Adler's 1907 theory that those with anxieties have an "organic" predisposition to it and thoughts on psychologist Otto Rank's 1926 theory of birth trauma.

To Rank, birth was a trauma that served as the source for all future anxiety. Freud disagreed. He concurred that the moment of birth is a crisis and an infant's first experience of danger and that the infant's response to birth is a kind of primal anxiety. However, he disputed Rank's claim that in that moment the infant suffered a "trauma" that is the model for all subsequent experiences of threat. He saw no evidence that infants receive from birth sensory impressions that they retain as traumatic memories or that those with difficult births are more likely than others to become anxiety prone. In contrast with Rank, he found it implausible to relate a child's fear of small animals—the kinds that burrow into holes in the ground—to his memory of emerging from the mother's womb, an event he could neither see nor conceptually comprehend. Furthermore, Freud believed that many childhood fears, such as those of being left alone in the dark or with an unknown person, point to a more logical definition of anxiety as simply a reaction to "helplessness in the face of a need."

In Freud's view, birth is the original moment of separation, when the child first parts from the mother. It is only gradually that the infant develops the faculties with which to distinguish itself from this "object" to which it once belonged and to appeal consciously to it when hungry or uncomfortable. At first the appeal is not directed to anyone at all. Over time the infant associates the presence of the mother or other familiar caregiver with the satisfaction of its needs and, when left alone or in the company of a stranger, reacts with anxiety at its helplessness. In expressing this, the infant employs the same physical anxiety response it showed at birth. It cries.

There have now been many studies investigating the influence of prenatal experience on the developing fetus, including studies of prenatal trauma. Perhaps, were he alive today, Freud would continue to refine his views on the idea of birth trauma or even prenatal trauma. But it is unlikely that he would revise his basic insight, which is that childhood and adult phobias can be due not only to external events but also to internal ones. A number of Freud's patients came to him with extreme phobias that, it seemed to him, bore only a tangential relationship to events that had occurred to them. He believed that the traumas behind these phobias were conflicts inside their psyches, conflicts treated as "dangers" no less than if they had been tigers in a forest. He posited that in each case the conflict could be related to specific dangers to the "ego" of the patient. His view on phobias was that they maintained anxiety created by the deeper conflicts, while disarming them of their true power, by substituting imagined dangers for the real ones. He likened this "defensive process" to the "flight" of the ego itself from a threat.

Freud drew his model of the human mind from the rest of nature. He saw the mind as an arena in which forces and energies competed for dominance. To Freud, emotions and impulses and wishes that were unconsciously rejected as unpalatable did not disappear but simply found other means of expression. An unseen conflict between an impulse and its conscious denial could be likened to the pressures building up between abutting tectonic plates underneath the earth's surface. Mental disorders would then be the earthquakes and volcanoes that released the slowly mounting tensions that had accumulated below.

Since fear is a protective response to external dangers, phobias, Freud reasoned, could be a self-generated response to, or representation of, an internal danger. Just as a person flees from danger in life, so in his mind he could flee from frightening thoughts by reexpressing them as fears of external objects and circumstances. A phobia could be channeling anxieties away from emotions, ideas, or memories too difficult to confront directly. Thus it followed that phobias could potentially be cured by seeking out their root cause.

One of the theories that made Freud's work so controversial in his day was the notion that sexuality flowered in the first five years of life and was then interrupted, to reemerge later, at the onset of puberty. This was by no means a concept original to Freud, but it has stuck to him the way the concept of evolution stuck to Darwin. In Freud's view, infantile sexuality is focused on the parent of the opposite sex, while when it resumes its course, it becomes generalized. Freud saw the desire of a small boy to be with his mother as automatically setting up a conflict with his father. In a sense, wrote Freud, all danger to the ego involves separation of a kind, starting with the separation of birth itself and culminating in the threat to the ego posed by death, the separation of the organism from life. In between, one faces what he called castration anxiety, separation from one's genitals (which he argued applies to women as much as to men) as well as, later in normal maturity, moral anxiety, the threat of disapproval from one's own superego, or conscience, a kind of rupture of the ego from the (self)-approval of the superego.

Again using a biological/Darwinian model for his theories, Freud found that just as sexual differentiation occurs only at a certain point in the developing fetus, so children pass through different stages that recollect earlier evolutionary forms of sexuality. While we delight in our feces at the age of two, an anal phase that recalls the time when creatures walked on all fours and their sense of smell was closer to the ground, we later tend to feel a mixture of disgust and some residual fascination with the whole excretory process. Sexual conflicts and dangers specific to the various stages of life normally lose their significance as one matures. However, said Freud, many adults have not resolved their original conflicts and, despite the fact that they can satisfy their own needs perfectly well, revert to a state of infantile helplessness when anxious, behaving "as if the old danger-situations still existed."

It wasn't because Freud himself was obsessed with sex that he emphasized its importance as an underlying human drive. It was because he was a biologist. From a biologist's viewpoint, the two most basic forces at work in an organism are reproduction and the will to survive, sex and eating.

If in outlining the stages of childhood development, Freud described its pleasures and physical gratifications as sexual, not sensual, it was simply to reduce forces down to their essence. Freud's models were in the physical and biological world. Just as the facial expression of disgust is a remnant of the physical action of vomiting—of getting rid of and rejecting whatever is toxic—so the transient pleasures of the senses flow like streams back to the ocean of our deepest needs. The nursing child derives physical pleasure, psychological security, and physical sustenance from its mother. Freud points out that the metaphor of eating is preserved in our language of love, when we speak of an "appetizing" love object and call our mates "honey" and "sweetie." The skin remains an organ of both love and sustenance. The caresses we received as infants and continue to seek in more mature forms later may help us survive. (More recently the French psychoanalyst Didier Anzieu has written about the "skin ego" [le moi-peau] and the importance of being caressed, calling physical affection an essential reinforcement of self.)

Freud saw phobias as among those psychological manifestations of inner sexual conflicts that could be cleared up if they were brought to the surface. Although he originally considered the repression of the conflicts to be the cause of the anxiety expressed in phobias, he later revised his view, stating that it was anxiety that caused the repression and the construction of a defense mechanism. Today we may not agree with him that "neurotic anxiety is transformed sexual libido," but his insight that anxiety symptoms often signal concealment—repression—remains convincing.

The beauty of his adoption of the story of Oedipus to frame his most famous complex is precisely that the underlying cause of the plague Oedipus tries to extirpate is within him. In just this way we may often find that we are trying in good faith to be rid of difficulties that we ourselves have constructed with equal energy. Like the "victims" of hysterical paralysis, we are the architects of our own handicaps.

Freud's one major case study of phobia was of Little Hans, a five-year-old boy. Hans's father was a music critic named Max Graf, an admirer and disciple of Freud's who kept a detailed journal about his son. (His identity was of course concealed in the published study.)

Hans had developed a morbid terror of horses, which made him dread going outside for fear that he would be bitten by one. He acquired his fear after seeing a horse carrying a heavy van suddenly fall in the street and make a ruckus, snorting and desperately kicking its legs. This phobia might have presaged general agoraphobia in the child since in early twentieth-century Vienna a fear of encountering horses was as inconvenient as a fear of encountering cars would be today.

Although Freud agreed with Darwin's speculation that many common childhood fears, including those of animals, are evolutionary remnants of responses to real threats, he brought his entire range of theories to bear on Hans's case, considering the fear and the moment Hans acquired it, in light of his interpretations of a child's sexual development.

The analysis in Freud's account hinges on an almost bewildering array of factors. Hans slept in the same room with his parents until he was almost four. When the father was away, he could sleep with his mother, sometimes imagining that he was the father. His fear of horses gradually developed during the period when his mother was pregnant and gave birth to his sister and he was moved into his own room. It became accentuated after he had stayed home for two weeks with influenza, after which he was particularly frightened to leave home for fear of encountering a horse.

What is striking in Freud's and the father's account is that pleasure, excitement, and fright are equally mixed in Little Hans's preoccupations from this time of his life. Hans loved his father but was also in competition with him for his mother's attention. In Freud's opinion, Hans was trying to sort out momentous matters: the workings of the body, the differences between the sexes, the distinctions between animals and humans, the way babies are produced, and other issues.

At the same time he was trying to adjust to sharing both his parents with a new sibling. The cheerfully inquisitive boy was fascinated by genitals ("widdlers," in the English Strachey's translation) and bowel movements ("lumpf")—his own, his father's, his mother's, his aunt's, the nursemaid's, his friends', and those of the animals he saw on the street or in picture books. While his mother warned him not to touch himself and even told him that he risked having his "widdler" "cut off" if he did so, she maintained the fictions of the day about sex and pregnancy, saying that "a stork" had brought Hans's sister. Meanwhile Hans had naturally observed the transformations she underwent during her pregnancy. Just after the birth Hans saw the bloody basins and vessels lying near her bed and even commented, "But blood doesn't come out of my widdler."

During the period of his fear (which he later recalled as "my nonsense"), Hans had a series of erotic dreams about his mother and other female figures that seemed both to stir him and to scare him. They served as the pretext for his getting into bed with his mother because he was frightened.

In Freud's account Hans feared being punished for his feelings and impulses: for sometimes wishing his father were out of the way, which he then couldn't reconcile with his fear of losing him; for wishing his sister had never been born and that his mother would not have any other children. He was frightened by the changes occurring in his family structure and was simultaneously trying to cope with his parents' admonitions about sexual expression, not to mention their dishonesty about reproduction.

In the end Hans's phobia had the effect of acting as an outlet for his anguish and drawing his parents' attention to it. At the same time, distressing as it was, it kept him at home, close to both his parents. Today we would call this "secondary gain."

Because Hans was introduced to "Professor" Freud and knew that his father reported their conversations to him, talking with his father brought with it a double reward. The conversations created a new bond, reassuring him that he hadn't lost his father as a result of having hostile feelings toward him and in the process compensated for the loss of his mother's attention. In addition, he was able to "work through," to use modern parlance, his unexpressed feelings with him. For example, he was able to narrate to his father how his sister had been brought by the stork and that he was fond of her but that he wished his mother would drop her in the bathtub and that she would die because she screamed so loudly. When the father said that "a good boy doesn't wish that sort of thing," the astute Hans answered, "But he may think it. . . . If he thinks it, it is good all the same, because you can write it to the professor."

In Freud's study, the falling horse came to stand, at various points, for Hans, the father, the mother, even the baby sister. Hans had himself played at being a horse and had himself had tantrums in which he fell down and "kicked his legs." He had also played horse with his father. He was frightened of horses' "black things" around their face—their blinders and the dark bits in their teeth—which Freud thought reminded Hans of his father's glasses and mustache. When the horse fell, it was as if his father had died. Hans feared that he would be bitten—that part of him would be cut off—like the punishment threatened by his mother. He feared the horse as an avenging force, with its own big "widdler," a force standing in for the father, outraged by his hostile feelings and his sexual excitement about his mother. The horse had also dragged a van behind it, in the way Hans's pregnant mother had carried the burden of her child, and had kicked its feet in its struggle, like a mother in childbirth. If the horse were the pregnant mother and fell, perhaps she would lose the child.

This is a mere suggestion of the many ways the symbolism of the horse is viewed in Freud's intricate study.

As his phobia diminished, Hans began to incorporate all its elements into his play. A crucial element in his cure occurred when he finally extracted from his father a realistic explanation of where children come from, thereby reassuring himself that both his parents had played a role in his own birth and that he still truly belonged to both of them. From this point on he began to fantasize that a number of his little friends were his own children, announcing to his father that he imagined he had created them by making "lumpf." Reminded that "boys couldn't have children," Hans explained that he was the father, that "Mummy" was the mother, and that in fact "Daddy" was now the grandfather, married to "Grandmamma" (i.e., the father's mother). This imagined ideal solution in which all family members had what they presumably wanted, while retaining one another, signaled the moment at which Hans was no longer afraid to go outside. The warring forces within him, which had found some analogue in the violence of the horse's struggle, were sufficiently resolved for him to let go of his fearful vigilance and move forward in his life.

Freud's extensive analysis examines a crossroads in the mind where pleasure, fear, and curiosity about life meet. It has at its foundation the burgeoning sexual desires of the young Hans and the difficulty he has sorting out what he can safely do and not do.

Admittedly this 1909 essay makes a strange entry point into Freud's writings. Freud met his subject only once before writing the account and was, in a sense, peripheral to the treatment reported in it. He had only advised Hans's father on what therapeutic approach to take and wrote his analytical study incorporating and interpreting the father's notes. There are many themes enmeshed in Hans's story. If by the end Hans is indeed cured, one can't help being skeptical about the reasons given for his recovery. Can guiding a five-year-old toward the expression of his inner conflicts actually purge him of neurotic symptoms?

Yet one comes away from the story of Little Hans with insight into how complex our adjustment to life changes must truly be and with a real feeling for the kind of inner dialogue that takes place beneath conscious thought. Freud recognized that Hans's phobia was constructed on top of an evolutionarily primed wariness about animals, but he saw it as Hans's outlet for the conflicted longings and fears of punishment he hadn't been able to express in other ways. Freud's genius revealed that the infinite resourcefulness of the human mind necessitates a greatly expanded concept of what can constitute "danger." The fear mechanism constructed for tigers in the forest can be used by humans to fight tigers in the mind. Indeed the entire fear apparatus itself can be appropriated by one side of the mind to combat another side. Thus we can be at war with ourselves, wrestling with a terror that is in fact also serving us as a defense.

Thirteen years after the successful "treatment," when Freud encountered Little Hans again, the boy had become a well-adjusted young man who had no memory whatsoever of his childhood fear.

Freud tried to cut through the skin of our shame and reticence to see what animates us. Yet far from having as his ultimate goal a hedonistic shucking off of civilization's restraint, he sought to understand the forces within us so that we could preserve what is best in us and neutralize those inner conflicts that make us susceptible to illness or capable of brutality. As someone who lived in the compartmentalized society of turn-of-the-century Vienna then witnessed the First World War and the rise of Hitler, Freud saw the urgency in studying the elemental forces of each individual mind.

Some of Freud's writings might seem dated today because they are, at first glance, hard to integrate with current insights into genetics and the brain. (Just where *is* the ego located, or the superego? Is there a cluster of brain systems that band together to form the Oedipus complex? When "feelings" are "repressed," where do they go?) In addition, psychological terminology itself has changed. While the words "neurosis" and "neurotic" persist in the general parlance, and "neurotic disorder" is used as a descriptive term in psychiatry, the Freudian "neuroses" have been replaced with diagnoses of specific disorders (anxiety, obsessive-compulsive, etc.) Three distinct categories of disorders—conversion disorder, dissociative disorder, and factitious disorder—now encompass the various aspects of what Breuer and Freud considered a single syndrome, hysteria. Someone described as neurasthenic in Freud's time would today be considered to be suffering from a somatoform disorder, a disorder characterized by physical symptoms that cannot be explained organically.

If Freud's account of the unraveling of phobias through the retracing of their origins may now seem overly optimistic, equally absurd, in many cases, is the idea that simply "unlearning" them while ignoring their significance will be efficacious. Some phobias may be annoying habits that indeed can be swiftly discarded in just a few sessions with a cognitive behavioral therapist. But in other cases they are part of a psychological continuum and of the person's way of life for a reason. Just as the obese woman with the eating compulsion is not necessarily cured by an intestinal bypass—indeed she may be confronted by the underlying emotional cause of her compulsion—so a person hampered by fears may not be free of them just because their surrogates are unmasked.

Looked at in a Freudian spirit, phobias could be viewed as a kind of discharge of fear in a safe place, a projection onto "neutral" or onto "evolutionarily primed" territory—onto things that can't really hurt you—of fears and memories, impulses and their consequences you don't want to confront. The phobia might be just a metaphor, a story you tell yourself to mask the real story. Does this process start with the repressed thoughts themselves or with a nervous system that is wound so tightly it generates fearfulness and attaches symbolic meanings to things?

If phobias can be considered safe and neutral, they are not the only example of the displaced, "safe" release of emotions. The most obvious example of such an outlet is in our dreams, where we can express ourselves in an unencumbered way precisely because we can disguise our meaning as much as we need to. But in fact most of our waking activities are exercises in sublimation. Playing contact sports discharges aggression; think of the Darwinian physical gestures and physical systems being deployed in boxing or in football. And all art is, in a sense, a waking dream. It allows the cortical ice to crack, and a river of feelings to flow through us, precisely because we are focused on representations and abstractions and not on the original sources of our emotions. We spend so much of our time trying to keep ourselves in order that our emotions need to find unexpected opportunities to release themselves, ways that won't cause too much disruption.

Our sexual energies are particularly devious about expressing themselves. How often sexual longing can be at its most powerful precisely when it will lead nowhere. I felt this way only the other day when I had an ear appointment. The audiologist testing me was a beautiful woman. When I was put in the soundproof chamber and saw her across from me through the pane of thick glass, sending me sound impulses through my headset, I was overwhelmed with longing for her. In this "safe" circumstance, I imagined myself irresistible and felt that if only the obstacles between us were removed, the young woman and I would be making passionate love. I could feel myself about to spring forward and leap through the glass barrier. In actuality, and sadly, it was probably the presence of the barrier that stimulated me to feel the "motion" embedded in the "emotion" of lust. In the solitude of having my ears checked, my mind sought relief from its fears of aging and decline and tried to mitigate them with comforting thoughts of rapturous union with the audiologist. This is no doubt what a shipboard romance or a passing crush usually is: a distraction, a way to improve an experience or merely to feel better, a safety valve. Unlike feelings of love, a crush tends to evaporate when we are removed from the context in which it occurs.

There is a law of competing stimuli. One can scientifically measure the exact degree of mitigation one stimulus effects over another. When we instinctively grip the dentist's chair while having a cavity filled, the sensation of pressure against our hands measurably lessens the pain we are feeling in our teeth. In a sense, the same principle was at work, from an emotional point of view, when I was having my ears tested. I instinctively added a positive feeling into an emotional mix that was preponderantly negative. I was trying to counteract the emotional pain.

What about competing *negative* stimuli? Who is to say if, in a similar way, we aren't making use of mice, bats, snakes, ghosts, tunnels, bridges, or blood to counterbalance deeper dreads and turn them into safely avoidable forms, seeking relief from their true meaning? If our fears are often drawn from a predictable repertoire of stimuli, does that contradict their individual usefulness?

Freud sought to map the forces at work behind and within our subjective experience. He tried to discern patterns that would hold true for humanity generally. In this endeavor he tried to maintain his objectivity and rationality as a scientist, attempting to factor out his own biases. As he wrote to Carl Jung, he was above all wary of "occultism." He regarded his work as science, as rigorously scientific deduction from evidence, subject to continual revision as observation warranted, not as some kind of speculative philosophy. In *Inhibitions, Symptoms and Anxiety* he stated: "We all know well enough how little light science has so far been able to throw on the problems that surround us. But however much ado the philosophers make they cannot alter the situation. Only patient, persevering research, in which everything is subordinated to the one requirement of certainty, can gradually bring about a change. The benighted traveler may sing aloud in the dark to deny his own fears; but, for all that, he will not see an inch further than his nose."

If today Freud is criticized for describing the life of the mind in "metaphorical" terms, in what terms should it be described? That the patterns in our mental life can be explained does not mean that they can be adequately expressed in terms of our DNA or the "electrical impulses" in the brain. The resonances stirred by the dialogue between brain systems, between the brain and the rest of the human organism, between the old brain and the new brain, between the human organism and the world in which it lives, create an inner music that may turn out to be discussable only through metaphor and art. We have physical evidence of the mind's patterns and of the effects of different chemicals on these patterns. But the music of the mind, the way it sounds from its inner orchestra of its billions of neurons, in which the tensions between what creatures used to be and what we now are, between our vulnerabilities and our need to survive, between our infantile wishes and the demands of adult life, between our memories and our present perceptions, between our desires, fears, disgusts, and rationality, can be deduced only from what we humans report and by what we manifest in our bodies and behaviors.

Is this perhaps what Freud meant when he spoke of the doctrine of behaviorism as a psychology constructed without consideration of the phenomenon of consciousness itself? He wrote of psychoanalysis, a term he coined and whose literal meaning is "soul analysis," that the "starting-point of this investigation is provided by a fact without parallel, which defies all explanation or description—the fact of consciousness."

Freud had to fight to demonstrate the complexity of our inner lives. Today's pharmacological age tends to gloss over it, reducing everything to chemistry and leaving the impression that the internal issues Freud said we wrestled with don't really matter very much and don't necessarily need to be "resolved" in order for us to feel well. Freud's writings provide a corrective to such glibness. His depth of investigation reminds us of the infinite resonance of our thought processes and of our relationships: to our parents, our siblings, our mates; the darkly primal significance of our simplest activities: our micturitions and defecations, our sexual experiences, the minute details of our physical behavior. Freud's observations, like those of Darwin, kindle a sense of awe at how even our most trivial experiences reach infinitely backward and forward in time.

It is interesting to read Freud alongside current texts confidently detailing the neurological underpinnings of mental life. Despite the fact that much of what Freud wrote might seem intriguingly compatible with current neurological science (one thinks of the conflicts between the emotional worlds of the two halves of the brain, for example, or the notion that the limbic system could be seen as a kind of id), new books on the brain are often almost mockingly dismissive in their references to Freud. Here is Rita Carter on Freud's explanation of phobias, in her lucid, instructive *Mapping the Mind*: "Freud maintained that irrational fears arose because the feared object had come to symbolize something that really was frightening but that was for some reason too embarrassing or awful to acknowledge. . . . Explanations such as this have now, at last, been shown to be ludicrously elaborate. Phobias can be produced by manipulating quick basic brain mechanisms—there is no need to involve sophisticated cognitive machinations like symbolism, guilt and covert desire." Perhaps. But Freud brought to his observations of people the kind of Darwinian respect for the interconnectedness of things that we need if we are to understand what is happening inside neuroanatomy. One needn't be a Cartesian dualist to feel that knowing the mechanics of the brain doesn't preclude the continued need for theories of the "mind."

It is interesting to compare Freud's reference to a mother playing peekaboo with her child with Carter's. Freud's account hinges on elemental forces of sex and survival and describes the learning of fundamental concepts and emotional lessons, Carter's on the activation of the brain system responsible for spatial awareness occurring during the period when such games are played. Both passages are informative, but not in the same way.

Carter has written: "As the baby gets older mylenization creeps outward and brings increasing numbers of brain areas 'on-line.' The parietal cortex starts to work fairly soon, making babies intuitively aware of the fundamental spatial qualities of the world. Peekaboo games are endlessly intriguing once this part of the brain is working because babies then know that faces cannot really disappear behind hands—yet the brain modules that will one day allow them to know why have not yet matured."

Freud's description of peekaboo, which follows, first detailed many ways in which the child, who in the womb has been part of the mother and who later, once born, is entirely dependent upon her, gradually learns that she is actually a separate being. At first, in the face of any separation from her, the child experiences what can only be a ghastly anguish: "As soon as it loses sight of its mother it behaves as if it were never going to see her again: and repeated consoling experiences to the contrary are necessary before it learns that her disappearance is usually followed by her reappearance. Its mother encourages this piece of knowledge which is so vital to it by playing the familiar game of hiding her face from it with her hands and then, to its joy, uncovering it again. In these circumstances it can, as it were, feel longing unaccompanied by despair."

Many of the principles Freud explored seem neurologically confirmed today: the idea that buried emotions can build up, accumulating tension; the notion of checks and balances between impulses and restraints; the intertwined relationship between physical sensations and thoughts; the indelible imprint of the first years of life. Furthermore, the idea of free association still constitutes the only known way to get even a glimpse of the vast web of thought that may be entangled in a single perception, a single instant of mental activity. The mind's density is such that only patient archaeology can lead to the separating out of some forgotten memory or parental voice or bizarre linkage of associations in what we "feel" at a given moment.

Most centrally, Freud's insight that we carry our past inside us as a permanent present seems completely, physiologically factual. The distant past accrues innumerable new meanings and connections through the experiences of intervening years, but inside us the past is still *there*, as if it were occurring now. As memoirist Anne Thackeray Ritchie wrote in 1894, "There is often a great deal more of the past in the future than there was in the past itself at the time . . . one learns little by little that a thing is not over because it is not happening with noise and shape and outward sign." No matter how old and jaded we have become, how long our parents have been dead, or how far we have traveled from their world, inside we are still waiting for our mother to come and kiss us good night, holding our ears from angry outbursts, cowering from being struck, or are hoping to be rewarded for eating our vegetables with a warm hug.

Chapter Ten

Change and Trauma

Home is where one starts from. As we grow older
The world becomes stranger, the pattern more complicated
Of dead and living. Not the intense moment
Isolated, with no before and after,
But a lifetime burning in every moment
And not the lifetime of one man only
But of old stones that cannot be deciphered.
—T. S. ELIOT, "EAST COKER"

The year my sister Mary left home for good, 1956, was probably the most difficult year of my early life, but I didn't know it at the time, and I don't remember the year very well. I remember only vaguely the moment when I realized that she was not returning. If separation anxiety could be manufactured in an instant by one event, this would have been its genesis. But the separation anxiety was one-, two-, or even threefold. Mary's unforeseen disappearance created what must have been a terrible constellation of emotions: grief, loneliness, guilt, bewilderment, rage, disillusionment, shock, the sense of having been betrayed by my parents, and perhaps also relief. I went from being a twin to being, to all appearances, not a twin at all. We went from being a family with two females and three males in it, to being one comprising one female and three males. I was now separated from Mary and had, in a way, a new beginning, as if there had never been a Mary. This created a sensation of falseness about my circumstances that I feel to this day, alongside an ingrained sense of culpability. Additionally, there must have been tremendous fear.

Mary's "exile" demonstrated that one could be turned out of the house for being too difficult to handle or understand, for being too inefficient mentally, or for being too wild. This added yet another layer of mystification to an already fairly mystifying atmosphere. It turned out that even in our temperate environment something extremely violent could occur. Since as far as I can remember, her departure wasn't discussed at any length and certainly wasn't ever described as some sort of cataclysm, the sense of violence gave teeth to every unstated rule and every pleasant expectation in our family life. I am sure that I feared for myself and also for my brother, while never consciously thinking that Mary had been punished. Nothing would have surprised my parents more than the notion that their silence on the subject only made matters worse. They must have agonized over their decision, and it must have been hard for them to move forward with their lives after making it. In a way they lost Mary twice, first as the normal child they had expected and later as the daughter who lived with them.

As far as I can recall, it happened in this way. Having had no success trying to get Mary to adjust to schools in New York, my parents were pleased when they heard of a summer camp in Cape Cod being started by a woman psychologist, a specialist in the field of retarded children. The "camp" was really just a big, sprawling house made of the gray clapboard often used in that area, in a beautiful spot on the water, with a jungle gym and swings out front and a sandy beach not far away. There would be only about thirteen children there, all of them with mental problems of one kind or another. I can't remember specifically the drive to visit the camp with Mary or the drive to drop her off there, but I assume we did both as a family group. I certainly remember visiting later. Mary was able to run around freely there and was also instructed in reading and in arithmetic in a new way that seemed to be working. The camp was called Sandpiper, after the local bird.

At the end of the summer my parents told my brother and me that the camp director had decided to turn Sandpiper into a school and that Mary would stay there. From then on we visited her several times a year for two hours or so, but she never returned home. Ten years later the school closed, and Mary was taken to the institution in Delaware where she still lives. At first we took yearly trips to visit her, but after my father's heart attack these became her yearly visits to see us. She would be brought by a member of the staff from the institution, have a birthday lunch, and leave. For me, these were happy occasions and gave me the sensation of a window opening. When I was in my teens and twenties, I often suggested going to visit Mary by myself. My mother discouraged this. Not wishing to upset her, I didn't press the point. Eventually her prohibition became my own. I never went there. My agoraphobia and some inner obstruction had made the trip to see my own twin begin to seem like a danger-ous trek across the desert.

I don't truly recall the discussion about Mary's remaining at the camp. I don't remember any discussion, and I don't remem-ber saying anything or asking anything about it at the time. When I try to think about it, I remember nothing except a kind of pulsating blankness.

At around this same time, the fall, winter, and spring follow-ing my eighth birthday and continuing into my fourth-grade year, I experienced a number of other smaller shocks. They left me even more susceptible to anxiety, but without any way to understand my feelings or communicate them. Despite my father's example, I didn't know what anxiety was.

In third grade my home room teacher was a young woman, gentle, blond, and attractive Miss Frost. This is about all I can clearly recall about her: Being in the classroom with her felt good, and she was tender and quiet when you went over to her desk and she explained something to you personally.

Over Thanksgiving holiday she died. My mother received a phone call from the school saying that Miss Frost had been suffering from headaches and had gone to a doctor. While in the waiting room she'd felt unwell, had gone over to the window, opened it, become dizzy, and fallen out to her death. At the very same time her fiancé was also "in the air," in an airplane flying from a foreign country—I forget which—to join her and get married.

When I received this news, I was in the living room with my brother. I remember that I was goofing around when our mother appeared, looking sad, and told us the story. After digesting this for a moment, my brother (then thirteen) proposed a game of chess. "Life goes on," he said.

The dim realization that the story of Miss Frost's death had possibly been altered hovered over me. I began to dream of her frequently, with images of falling, of her boyfriend flying, and of her face looking anguished. She always appeared with her blond hair slightly disheveled, with wisps floating away from her head, as if she were flying. She looked haunted by something and in several of the dreams put up a finger and warned me with the words "Three years. Three years." In one dream she had my father's face with her hair; in another she had the face of the sister of our housekeeper Bessie (a woman who, like my own sister, had an abnormality, an unusual skin pigmentation). These dreams terrified me. Sometimes when they happened, I would run into my parents' bedroom and soak up the comfort of their warmth and nighttime smells, smells I now recognize in the middle of the night in my adult self. Both of them would wake up and never seemed to mind. It was always my father's job to tell me clearly that "it was just a dream."

I had already started suffering from a fear of the dark, so common in children of that age, a common transient tendency that, it would appear, is really the fear of one's own imagination, so fertile and developing so exponentially at that time. You fear what you might *imagine* in the dark. In the dark everything you have begun to understand about life, everything you have held at bay in the light, comes floating to the surface. When you are a child, the moment you enter a darkened room, the tiredness of night and the spotted, febrile look of things seen through shrouds can come over you even if it is daytime outside and you are wide awake. Just as with a phobia, the fact that you are aware that the problem is imagined doesn't necessarily relieve you. My brother used to exploit this fear from time to time by asking me to go get something down the hall in a dark room and then laughing when I begged him to turn on the light.

Naturally such visions happen all the more easily when you are tired and in bed, trying to fall asleep. The distinctions between dreaming and seeing, or between what might actually be possible and what couldn't possibly happen, are far from clear even to adults, let alone to children. Traumas, like the disappearance of my sister or the death of my teacher or even things you only hear about or see a glimpse of as a child, are in part learning experiences that teach you hard lessons about just how bad things can get.

At around this same time I had an unsettling experience with a girl who lived in our building. We were playing catch in the dark alleyway next to the service entrance when a slack-jawed, befuddled-looking man appeared and started listlessly to follow my friend. After a moment I realized that he was holding something that looked like a hot dog in front of his trousers. It took me longer to register that it was his penis, or at least I realized it *had* to be. At first I froze; then I felt like running out of the alley and leaving both of them there; finally I yelled and gave the man a push, and he ran away, without even zipping up his pants. The entire incident surely lasted no more than a minute with only my shout breaking the silence. For several years after it, I would refer to "the hot dog man" and the fact that he had seemed both threatening and mentally unbalanced or, perhaps, like my sister, retarded, stayed with me. When I rushed upstairs to tell my mother, who was in laughing conversation on the phone, and had told her breathlessly that I had just seen an "attempted rape," she didn't put down the phone or change her tone until the call was over. I remember having a bitter feeling that she didn't believe that terrible things could be real or that even when they were, social equanimity should be maintained nonetheless. Later my father went with me to the police station, where they filled out a report about the incident and we met with a detective who showed us pictures of sexual criminals.

Afterward I developed a strange fear of a picture of a man in a cowboy hat on the front of a cereal box. He was a beefy-faced actor who played a sidekick in a TV western that I watched. There was something about his leering, dim-witted expression in the picture that scared me, and my brother used to chase me holding the cereal box in front of him, taunting me, calling out, "The man in the box! The man in the box!" If in fact the picture reminded me of the "hot dog man," I did not know it. Yet precisely that lack of awareness may have invested the face with its peculiar power over me. The emotional impact of this "attempted rape" had barely registered. Nor at an age only slightly older than Freud's Hans could I comprehend the many associations it might have stirred.

Another incident occurred during a class recitation when I was nine years old. I was standing in a group, and we were reciting a passage from the Bible in unison. I think it was a passage from Exodus, a story in which *all* Jews were "leaving home." The teacher, Miss Wyeth, was the sternest at the school and one of the few who taught through intimidation. (In the first week of school she had held up my book report on *Mrs. Piggle-Wiggle* in front of the whole class as an example of bad handwriting.) When we stood together in recitation that day, I must have suffered what is called parade syndrome. I remember it today as if it had just happened. We were standing and speaking and looking at Miss Wyeth, and suddenly there were little ants in front of my eyes. I had a prickly sensation in my eyelids, and a wave of cold air seemed to start at my feet and pass through me all the way up to my face. Then it was dark. When I woke up, I was viewing Miss Wyeth and my classmates from below and they were peering down at me no longer reciting. I looked around and saw everyone's feet and realized that I was on the floor on my back with a slight pinching feeling in my forehead.

This fainting episode, which never recurred, left me uneasy whenever I had to stand for long periods of time, particularly in performing situations. I already suffered during chorus rehearsals, so performances, when we had to stand, became still worse. Then another incident added an unpleasant association to the idea of group singing. I can't remember whether it preceded or followed the fainting episode.

In addition to sometimes having acting roles in the yearly Christmas pageant, I always sang in the treble choir, which, robed in black and white, opened the pageant by marching down the aisles of the auditorium singing and then continued singing facing the audience. On the Sunday of the pageant during this same year, when I was crossing Park Avenue on the way to the performance, a tall, distinguished-looking elderly man approached me from the opposite side of the street. Unexpectedly he seemed to lose all his vitality and collapsed to the ground almost at my feet. His head landed squarely on the cement, and his hat—a fedora, not unlike my father's—fell to one side. He lay there, and I stood in front of him stark still. Then I ran and cried out, people started to gather, and a doorman called for an ambulance.

When I went upstairs to the rehearsal room, I was trembling, and my heart was pounding. My face was ice cold. From the window in the music room I could see the Park Avenue corner where the man was still lying in his coat, with a crowd around him, and it seemed a long time until the ambulance came. The school conductor looked out too and said he in fact knew the man, adding that perhaps he had had a heart attack or a stroke, or perhaps he had died; there was no way to tell. He laughed lightly, saying that I looked "as white as a sheet," that I shouldn't worry, the man would be taken care of, he might not even be dead. From the window I kept an eye out for what was happening on the corner. To me, the man did look dead. By performance time an ambulance had taken the man away. As I later walked down the aisle singing, I felt as if my legs had turned to lead. I felt as if I were at my own funeral.

I never learned what happened to the man who fell on the street. But his memory became a memory of *falling,* of sudden loss of self, mixed with memories of a teacher who had fallen to her death and of my own fainting episode, with its connection to leaving, "exodus."

Around this same time I began to feel sick in certain situations.

The physical reactions became as predictable as asthma attacks or allergies. For some reason, though, I never mentioned them to anyone—not to my best friends, my brother, or my parents. It is interesting, in view of Freud's perspective, that these "anxiety attacks" or "panic attacks" coincided to a degree with the onset of conscious sexual feelings, and it isn't too difficult to make a comparison between the general trajectory of accumulating panic and of accumulating sexual excitement. I remember sitting in assembly at school in the middle of the row, surrounded by my peers, perhaps two hundred or so of them, feeling the gradual spread of an inner tension that became increasingly intolerable. The tension would be centered in my stomach and would gradually increase to the level of extreme nausea, accompanied by a nagging nervous tightness in every muscle and a feeling of breathlessness, as if the valve that normally kept my breathing under control had suddenly lost its function. I would sink deeper and deeper into my chair, pinned there, isolated, and ashamed, as if singled out for torment. The experience would reach a climax and my face would become cold as if a winged ghost had passed over it. Bizarrely, these sensations were redoubled when we sang. The wondrously stirring chorus of voices would unhinge me and make me feel a sense of estrangement, as if I were surrounded by bellowing prehistoric creatures, and I needed to get out from under it, out of the hall, if possible, to get some air. Of course I wouldn't leave. I remained in a churning, sickening void—apart from reality—until the assembly was over.

I suffered from frequent stomachaches during this same period and also often cried myself to sleep, sometimes singing softly while crying, making myself cry with my own singing. I had a preoccupation with the Holocaust. I can't remember where the knowledge of this part of history came from or exactly when the preoccupation began, but I knew that we were Jews and that not long before "the Jews" had been rounded up and sent to concentration camps and killed. Somehow the notion of Mary's camp and the concentration camps that Jews were sent to became combined in my imagination. When I would lie awake before going to sleep, I would imagine my parents and my brother and me—but not Mary—rounded up and separated from one another and sent away and killed. I would picture us surrounded by throngs of frightened people being bullied by soldiers and picture my parents and my brother being roughly dragged off, waving good-bye, and I would cry.

Around the age of ten I began taking leadership roles in student government. Although it was a relief to stand up during large meetings—to escape, as it were, from being submerged in the crowd—I also suffered from anxiety when I tried to make my voice heard. When I stood to speak, I was shocked by the beating of my heart and by my shortness of breath.

I was deeply ashamed of my reactions when I was in the center of a row of students, part of a choir, occupying my chair playing clarinet in the middle of the school orchestra, or standing up to speak. But in a sense I didn't even know I had a problem. I simply came to expect these habitual physical reactions. I confessed them to no one. In my chair in orchestra I would feel better while playing the clarinet part, but during the rests in my part I would start to feel ill and would break out in a sweat, thinking of how it would look if I suddenly bolted from the stage.

While unconsciously absorbing his anxieties, I consciously imitated my father's work habits. On Sundays, I sometimes used to draw while he sat on the sofa in the living room in his bathrobe, working on his magazine proofs. He used to look up over his reading glasses and ask me how my "work" was going. Later he would give me old proofs to mark up and "edit," and I enjoyed crossing paragraphs out or writing "no good" or "terrible" next to them, while he edited for real. I also loved to hear him at the piano and sometimes sat underneath the instrument while he played. (His rhythmical foot against the pedal left a permanent hole in the rug.) I started playing the drums along with him, joined by my brother on the violin, but other than being able to keep a beat, I showed no particular musical aptitude.

By the end of my eighth year I discovered music for real. It happened at a ballet performance of *Swan Lake* at the old City Center. Near the end of the story, when the prince watched the swans disappearing off stage, and the music swelled into a peroration of its rhapsodic tune (nothing could be more "minor key" than that melody), I felt something overwhelming happen to me. Some lurching hidden tragic power coursed through me and made me shiver and feel that I had been living a very long time, as if clock time, chronological time, had no meaning. I felt old. The theater seemed to ascend to the stars with the music, and it was as if we all were remembering life from far away.

After that, when I heard my father playing his version of *Rhapsody in Blue*, I listened differently, with the aim of remembering what he was doing. I began to spend long hours at the piano trying to reconstruct the parts I liked and making up little phrases of my own. I bonded with the piano. It was as if I were in dialogue with it. Sometimes strange thoughts or individual words would get stuck in my mind while I experimented with different intervals and chords or played phrases repeatedly over and over. I remember that the word "divorce" was one of the words.

By the time I was ten I was putting short musical bits together and calling them pieces of music. One of the first was called "The Dying Accordion Player." My brother particularly encouraged me and, taking my new line of "work" seriously, immediately incorporated it in our puppet productions. I still couldn't read music very well, and I asked my parents if I could take piano lessons. That's how my composing started.

It is said that small children who lose their mothers sometimes huddle next to radiators for hours on end. In some ways I believe that the piano had become my twin, and I huddled close to it for warmth. The instrument connected me with both Mary and my father.

Interestingly, then, for one who later became a musician, music became associated in my mind with both release *and* entrapment, with both ecstasy *and* dread.

I see now that my early fear of the dark—the fear of what you might see in your mind when real images are removed—is uncannily like my adult fear of open space or of the blank sheet of fog on which one has no choice but to project images from within. I also carried with me into my teenage and college years a terror of death that came sweeping over me when the lights were turned out, until engulfed, I would start up in bed and turn the lights back on.

This began after my sister had left home, when I still slept in my childhood bed and watched, as I was falling asleep, the columns of light created by passing trucks and cars cross the ceiling again and again, and listened to the closing doors and sneezing sounds of the buses starting up after picking up passengers. The certainty that death would someday come, no matter what, and that *after that* I would never again return, never live again, forever, that I would be gone and never come back, and that this was going to happen and no one could stop it—this certainty would start just like my fainting, at my feet, and sweep up through my entire body until it overwhelmed me. It was mixed in with the certainty that my parents would be gone and that everyone would be gone and that no matter how many people kept living, they all would eventually be gone and that everything would be forgotten. Somehow, turning on the light and seeing the firmly etched outlines of the bedpost, and the lamp I had made in woodworking class, with its little bucket and the handle and chain in the form of the pump to a well, seemed reassuring. But when I turned the light off again, the certainty that there was no help, that my parents could not help me, and that there was no escape from the fact of it, not even some special hint of a way out that might just apply to me would return. So in a sense death was here *now*, we all were already living *in death*, and all life would someday be blotted out, never to be remembered. Such thoughts would again flood me in waves that increased in height and reached a peak, just like panic. But unlike panic, when the waves subsided, they left behind a silt of irrefutable truth.

At twelve I wanted to explode but couldn't. In the apartment in New York I was enveloped, almost enshrouded, by my parents' expectations, unwritten rules that had become internal constraints. The light streamed through the windows from Central Park, and my mother smiled brightly her red-lipsticked smile, yet the available air was stale and trembled from undisclosed blows. My parents seemed so gentle. Somehow there was no way to say what I felt, let alone scream it. Sexually I was bursting—I was twelve, after all—but as tightly curbed as a little monk. Beneath my sunniness there was also rage that my family was somehow a sham, that I was a twin who wasn't supposed to feel like one, that we were Jews with an Irish name. I felt that huge passions and angers that somehow couldn't be mentioned were seething within me and within the house and that the world was raw and crude but had to be referred to politely in perfect sentences. There were blinding hatreds in the air that couldn't be named; there was sex that couldn't be spoken of; there were deep mysteries that had to be sanitized and secularized; there was deep competitiveness and there were deep character flaws that couldn't be acknowledged. Life was big and wild and open and natural and unfathomable, but we were supposed to keep it orderly and routinized and closed and fixed. Beneath my smooth surface was a festering abscess that needed to be lanced and desires that wanted out.

At around the same age, when I was traveling with my parents in a chauffeured limousine after seeing my brother off to high school in Vermont, while my father sat next to me editing his manuscripts, I suddenly vomited. My parents weren't unduly upset, but I was. Motion sickness is common enough, particularly in childhood. But the moment left a shadow. In memory, the upset stomach became confused with the sights and sounds accompanying it: the way the sun glinted on the asphalt, the green of the highway divider, the whoosh of the cars.

I don't know what had happened on the morning of that trip. But away from the tightly monitored family cocoon of our apartment in New York City, I burst, if only metaphorically. The highway stretched onward and outward to the wide world, but we were in a confined space and, within that, hemmed in by slogans, rules, and rituals that could not even be identified as such. Perhaps there had been an argument between my parents and my brother, and I was scared that he would, like Mary, be permanently left behind. Perhaps, as happened so often, my father had stopped the car to make one of his frequent calls at a roadside telephone booth to "the magazine" (and often, to his other "wife"), creating the usual (if unacknowledged) anxiety in my mother. Perhaps my father's own dread of travel was palpable that morning. Perhaps being alone with my parents—with their pain, their tensions, their need to control and monitor each other— created a powerful force field that upset me. Or perhaps I passionately *needed* to be alone with them in order to express myself, and it had become impossible not to bring up what was inside. Perhaps here in this closed yet wide-open world my self-control collided with my imperative to live, to flee, to get out. Or perhaps I had simply eaten the wrong breakfast.

As creative as my home environment was, it was in equal measure repressive. As kind as it was, it was also unkind. I had to hold in many of my thoughts and my perceptions of much of what I saw. My father was an editor. When you vomit, you cannot choose, you cannot edit. When you are enraged, you cannot edit. In bringing up the contents of my stomach, I was letting out something that normally stays in. It was one of the few moments when alone with my parents, I lost control of what I was doing.

I never had a chance to come properly to terms with Mary. Though she was in some ways, more even than my mother, my first love, she was, at the same time, the cause of deep anxiety and fear. After her departure I was left with an unassuageable loneliness. The mysteriousness of her behavior when we were children, as well as the loss of her companionship at age eight, left me ill equipped to acknowledge my own quirks to others, let alone break out of my stabilizing family role, a role that I had assumed voluntarily and have continued to carry with me, I believe, into an adult context. Music gave me an enormous outlet but also protected me from being understood. In music I could be wild, aggressive, irreverent, and unpredictable; in life I shunned behaviors that would remind me of the chaos of Mary's mind. I tended to act like and feel like the soul of reasonableness—except when I was ambushed by my inner demons. This is still the case, and there is something false about it. My better, darker music represents something truer about me; it is way ahead of the rest of me. A Japanese psychiatrist who had only heard me described put it this way: "His music and his phobias are the same."

I never got over the suspicion that I caused Mary's birth trauma myself. After all, I was there, right next to her when it happened. At the very least, I assumed deep down, I must have experienced a bit of the trauma myself, and the damage would eventually be revealed. I think of this every year on my birthday.

After the summer when I was eight, I felt doubly guilty: guilty of whatever had happened at our birth that left me less harmed, and guilty that she had been banished. I wondered if I was the cause of both catastrophes. I feared the consequences of being out of control or of rebellion. I also feared the inner explosions that racked me when I was angry, sexually excited, or panicky, those eruptions of the autonomic nervous system that make all of us human. They must have reminded me of the seismic jolts that animated Mary so frighteningly.

At an early age I had been shocked by the fragility of the human mind, by seeing how close we all are to being unable to orient ourselves, sort things out, and think clearly. So most of all, I must have feared the confusion and weird disorientation of my panic attacks, those moments when the world would become so strange that I would feel as if my own mind and Mary's had merged.

Chapter Eleven

Agoraphobia

> Can it be that one day, off it goes on, that one day I simply stayed in, in where, instead of going out, in the old way, out to spend day and night as far away as possible, it wasn't far. Perhaps that is how it began. You think you are simply resting, the better to act when the time comes, or for no reason, and you soon find yourself powerless ever to do anything again. No matter how it happened.
> —Samuel Beckett, *The Unnamable*

As a child I subscribed to the *National Geographic* and collected maps, dreaming of travels and an international life as a musician and composer. I still brighten at the sight of foreign place-names and feel excitement hearing from foreign friends and strangers. I love the cadences of foreign languages and the sounds of unfamiliar music, like the irresistible twang of Chinese opera singers and the undulating buzz of the Indian sitar. I keep a map of Paris over my piano for inspiration. If I never backpacked or hitchhiked across the country as a teenager, as some of my friends did—that kind of improvisatory trek would have violated every maxim of my upbringing—I did enjoy being in nature and going on camping trips. Even now I love walking in the woods; I love imagining that I am miles from civilization. But I won't walk in very far, no more than maybe a half mile at most, just enough to be entirely enveloped and to experience the solitude. My ideal environment is one that appears to be rustic but is actually only moments from houses and stores. I stand at the edge of the woods, but I feel an extraordinary love for the darkness there and for the way the light gets parceled out, dappled, shafting through, around, and across the trees, and the way the old rotting trunks, sonorously crunchy underfoot, lie across the forest floor, collecting olive green moss and mushrooms of every shape, swarming with insect life. There is no sense of scale there, only many microworlds, created by the deep shadows and sudden patches of warm sun, captured on humps or dips of earth, on carpets of green-yellow lichen, or in the trembling streaks of a muddy brook. There are only the sounds of buzzing and calling and twittering and running water—the joy of no humans.

The agoraphobic predicament seems to be that one cannot easily move forward in the world without knowing already what lies ahead. Without making a conscious effort to fight the tendency, one can become increasingly stuck, avoiding even the *possibility* of a panic attack. One therefore tends to travel the road that one already knows and where one has previously felt fine. This restrictiveness is not necessarily reflected in every aspect of one's life. In fact, as with any handicap, the problem may be balanced by compensatory strengths. In my work and in my personal life I have not entirely clung to what was predictable or what has previously been done, although I have noted these inclinations in myself at times. I certainly don't need to keep repeating myself in my music, as I seem to in my traveling routes. The one moment in my life when I was particularly stuck in my work was when I was first becoming an out-and-out agoraphobe, in France studying music in the early 1970s. But as an adult composer I am disappointed when my music doesn't have enough of its own voice, disappointed when things I write don't break *some* new ground—at least in terms of what I myself have done. I love modern, current art, and I know that only when I feel some sense of danger and nakedness and newness in what I am writing is my work saying something individual enough to be of interest. I do seek surprise in music. In fact one critic introduced a review of my music with the headline MUSIC OF UNEXPECTED TWISTS AND TURNS. But my love of newness and freshness in art is not matched in daily life, where I tend to be wary of the unexpected.

When habits of avoidance and anxiety persist for a long time, they become a part of you, like chronic pain. The brain gets used to the connections, and they harden. Amazingly, though, even the adult brain can build entirely new connections. The old ones can become undone—if a person is ready to undo them—and eventually, with hard work, replaced. I am always surprised thinking about how my sense of safety has been transferred from New York to Vermont and how my feeling of being a fish out of water in Vermont gradually disappeared. Now I feel it when I go to New York. Still, it is a fact that with work, many people do unlearn agoraphobic patterns completely.

In order to be ready to change a habit as far-reaching as agoraphobia, one has to be motivated to change all that has grown customary *around* the phobic habits. One has to *want* to be less encumbered and perhaps be prepared to face the real anxieties lying in wait once the phobias are removed. It seems clear from the studies and successful treatments available in the last forty years that medicines and cognitive behavioral therapy can often be helpful in and of themselves as treatments. Certainly simply remembering one's childhood is unlikely to result in being cured of agoraphobia. However, it stands to reason that if phobias are getting seriously in a person's way, they may be shielding him as much from his inside world as from that outside. At the very least, he is living in dread of being left alone with panic and with all that he is thinking when he panics, with what panic *means* in his case. Just as, although we all are afraid to die, death actually has an infinite number of possible meanings, so panic, although physiologically uniform, is different in its significance for each person.

If phobias are decoys, what will strike us when the decoys are removed? What awaits us in the emptiness of space?

About fifteen years ago I had a bad bout of laryngitis. It made it hard for me to teach, but I kept going to work, and it kept returning, so in the end I had to stop teaching completely for many days, stop speaking on the phone, and write down everything I wanted to say on a big yellow pad. The problem lasted for several weeks, and I began to panic. Never once during that time did I think about how hard it had always been for me to speak up for myself, let alone to scream, as Mary screamed— not because it was "sensible" for her to, but because sometimes she had to scream. I can see now that my loss of voice mirrored my inability to speak.

When my children were small, there were some terrible mo-ments when they were in pain or simply distressed in some inner way and I couldn't make the problem stop. Sometimes they would wake up in a bad mood, or very tired, or with a cold, and they would search for a cause and look to me to solve the way they felt, as if I were in charge of all nature, the way I was in charge of paying the electricity bill. I remember their looks of reproach; they were still young enough to think that whatever happened to them was caused by their parents or could be alleviated by them. It was such a wonderful feeling to be able to give them a hug, or kiss them and smooth the hair from their forehead, or give them some cough syrup, and make them feel better. But sometimes there was nothing that I could do to truly help, because their bodies and minds were simply doing what they needed to, which was to feel bad.

We are born in denial. Like the pre-Copernicans of the Middle Ages, who thought that the earth was the center of the universe, we start by believing we are the center, that everything we see is but an extension of us, there to support us. It takes years for it to dawn on us that our parents merely participated in a process that they didn't understand any better than we do. They no more "made" us than they made themselves or the trees outside the window. They were made as we were made. Neither they nor we are the center. There is no center.

My parents didn't design their genes, or mine, or decide ahead of time that they would fashion five children, two of whom would die and one of whom would mystify them, or that the stresses of life would affect them this or that way, or that a truck driving too quickly across Amsterdam Avenue on a certain summer day in 1952 would happen to collide with a taxi carrying my mother. They didn't design my brother and me, and they didn't know that the environment of the camp my brother complained about in his letters home in summer 1957 was going to be rough and sadistic, and couldn't tell for sure if it would be better for his character development for him to learn to live through such a thing or for them to come and get him. (They eventually came and got him but only after an entire month had passed.) They didn't know if it would be better for me if they frequently reminded me that I was a twin, buying me books titled *You and Your Retarded Twin* or sending me to help out at Mary's school over summer vacation (as I in fact asked to do and was refused), or instead emphasized that I was a unique person and didn't need to feel "burdened" for my whole life by being Mary's twin. In retrospect, I think that shielding me didn't work well, but I do know that dealing with growing children is like being in a batting cage with ball after ball being thrown at you. You hit the balls you can. Amazingly, the score gets kept for a very long time.

I see now that holding down something as formative as having a twin is impossible. You can be *silent* about it, but you can't hold it down, and if you try, it will rebel inside you as surely as I rebelled against the muggers' attack in 1975.

In order to live reasonably fully, we first have to occupy our own skin; to remember and acknowledge, as much as possible, what actually happened, and to rage and scream about it, if need be. But then we face an endless chain of causes, and forgiveness settles in. Our parents were children who grew up and had their own children. And as Philip Larkin wrote:

> . . . they were fucked up in their turn
>   By fools in old-style hats and coats.

In the end we are alone with the responsibility of coping with our lives.

From the time Mary left the house until around the time I turned twenty-two, when I reached another critical juncture in my life, there were a number of things that I didn't enjoy doing, that caused me anxiety, but that didn't truly constitute agoraphobia. Children and young people simply don't have enough control over their lives to establish a general pattern of phobic avoidance. I usually felt anxious and sick on car and bus trips, but for many years I didn't pay much attention to where the bus was, whether on an open country road or a highway or passing through a tunnel. When I was around nine or ten, I enjoyed going to the top of the Empire State Building—at least twice—with my brother and looking through the "periscopes" at the splendor of Manhattan spread out below, having our picture taken, and, if I am not mistaken, making an instant recording of our voices in a recording booth. As a teenager at school in Vermont I enjoyed camping trips deep into the forest or up in the mountains. Up through college I didn't overly restrict myself on account of anticipated anxiety, taking subways, trains, and elevators despite the tension I felt and flying on planes several times, including on some fairly rickety ones. In 1968 I flew down to Washington with friends and stood in the middle of a crowd of half a million people in a march against the Vietnam War. I was panicky and asked my tall friend if I could sit on his shoulders, which I did; but at least I was there. On the return trip, for which we had rented a car, I had a terrible panic attack as we drove through the Holland Tunnel into New York City. Feeling a sense of suffocation, I tried to find relief by crouching in a ball on the floor of the passenger front seat until we had passed through back into daylight. My friend was very sympathetic. It was one of the last times I used such a route in traveling.

From a traditional Freudian point of view, I am well aware, some of my travel phobias—a car or train moving through a tunnel, the graceful liftoff of a plane, the experience of being at a great height—are sexually suggestive. I also know that I became increasingly agoraphobic at the very instant I began to emerge as an independent, sexually active man, following nature's directive to get out there, propagate, and learn to fly far from the nest. This was also the moment of true separation from my parents and from childhood, and although the memory of it was buried, separation anxiety had already marked me. My travel phobias escalated disastrously at a moment of rebellion and even disobedience in which, paradoxically, I risked being ostracized for choosing to leave. I had always feared banishment, and now that I was *choosing* to leave I wanted both to leave and *not* to, just as, no doubt, my parents may have wanted both things for me too. I wanted to know that I could always come back. I had always feared that once I had left, like Mary, I could never return. (". . . wasn't there a fork in the road back there at some point that I have already taken? How will I remember my way back?")

I also know that as an adult, perhaps like most people, I had conflicted feelings about sex. I absorbed both my father's intense desire for women and his unusual degree of shame about what people actually do with each other sexually. This has resulted in a checkered sexual history, with some highs and some extraordinarily bad lows. I have memories of happy, tender comminglings, alongside ones of depressing failure, where nothing felt natural and nothing worked properly.

For a young boy trying to figure out how to behave with women, being small and unconventional looking alters the dynamics of sexual experience. The same behavior that might pass as appealing masculine bravado if it came from someone more conventionally attractive gets regarded as rude or disgusting when issuing from someone deemed less desirable. And I felt guilty about my sexual feelings anyway. I didn't need any help thinking I was disgusting.

As a twelve-year-old I knew that "sex" and "love" were often traditionally linked, and was baffled to find my wild impulses stirred on a purely physical basis. The women portrayed in *Vogue* magazine, whose curved shapes, though encased in clothes, promised unheard-of ecstasies, didn't need to speak about their lives, thoughts, and feelings to inspire my excitement. This excitement certainly wasn't "love" and must have been something to be ashamed of instead. I actually wasn't sure what love was. My upstairs neighbor when I was eleven was a nice red-haired girl who let me kiss her on the lips from time to time and even wrote me notes signed "I Love You," but she was not my girlfriend. She was actually going out with the tallest boy in our class, someone who had nearly killed me in a tackle on the football field. There was another girl at school, Felicity, who had curly red (again) hair and freckles, with whom I had only a distant acquaintanceship. There was something about the sight of her pale, freckled, pudgy leg emerging from her skirt that stirred a smooth flow of honey within me and made me feel reckless. I reached for Felicity—to coin a phrase—and was rebuffed. Once at a party when I was ten or eleven, a beautiful girl took me aside and kissed me passionately, as romantic music played in the background. It had, in a way, no significance or consequences, but her warm breath on my face made me feel like a man.

Before I left for music camp at thirteen, my father told me that I might encounter an activity called masturbation while I was there, but he looked as if he might be about to commit suicide after our conversation. He did his best but actually communicated his own terror. I know now that he must have been afraid of handling it the wrong way and scarring me for life. He was incapable of saying, "I have done this myself"; it had to be "we" or "it" or "one" ("It's perfectly normal . . ."). In an effort to be tactful, he managed to imply that the concept of masturbation was sure to be new to me. This reinforced my shame about pleasures already taken. He communicated an impression that somehow the covered regions of the body, like its inner workings—and like distant areas of the world—were frightening.

How strange that so many of us act as if *Homo sapiens* were at first highly intelligent and then only later developed, much to his embarrassment, his animal traits. I am sure that if chimpanzees have such discussions as I had with my father, they are more straightforward ("Here's what you do . . ."). But perhaps this is precisely the point: It is because we began as "animals" that we now suffer shame, just as the teenager bridles when his mother strokes the back of his neck, because he remembers the times when he used to sit on her lap.

Not surprising, actual sex—as opposed to the idea that some people were "attractive"—was hard to mention in the family. I remember a discussion in which my brother brought up a memoir written by the father of one of his friends, the subject of which was a kind of international quest for sexual nirvana, a pilgrimage that took him to the Esalen Institute, I believe, and to India, to study the *Kama sutra*. The conversation simply stopped. My parents, usually so ready with commentary, became strangely speechless and flat, like radios lost between stations.

When I reached puberty, I was still so well behaved and young looking—at thirteen I looked about nine—that I felt expected to be innocent. This was reinforced in my family by my reputation for being impartial, controlled, and philosophical, not impulsive and carnal. (I already had a tendency to mirror people's expectations of me.) My first fantasies didn't get much beyond the notion of wrestling a girl to the ground and pressing against her soft flesh, yet even this seemed more like an act of aggression than like reasoned impartiality. I didn't quite know how to make a declaration to the world that I was a boiling caldron of sexual desire. I feared general mockery; I feared more rejections. Playing the part of Ariel in *The Tempest* when I was twelve, which I did all too credibly, helped cement my image as a kind of "sprite," as opposed to the dangerously attractive man I wished to be. I did not pass my early youth going from conquest to conquest, as some of my friends seemed to, but, as in my later travel patterns, encountered a series of inner prohibitions as well as outer ones, somehow restricting myself unconsciously even in how I presented myself. I hid behind the idea that I was small and therefore couldn't convincingly bring off a show of sexiness, but I now see that there are plenty of small Mick Jaggers in the world. I am now sure that for my own reasons, I simply didn't respond to those females who may have found my attributes acceptable ("Short guys are the *best!*"). I don't think that this side of my personality has completely changed to this day, despite all that has happened to me. For all my many "healthy" sexual impulses, most of which thankfully I have carried out at one time or other, I have never quite had the feeling that experiencing sex to the fullest extent, like experiencing life to the fullest extent, is a birthright.

It was years before I understood that sex was not just one thing, but rather a force that could be linked to many different emotions, activities, and associations. It could be solitary, in which case it could sometimes stir feelings of loneliness; it could apparently be communal (though not for me; I skipped all the group activities of the sixties); it could be straightforward, warm, and friendly; it could be an expression of the deepest connection between two people; it could be a merging directed toward making a child; it could be loving but disappointing; it could be alienated; it could be pleasurably convenient; it could be boring or unwanted; it could be a relaxed, joyful experience; it could be perverse; it could be heart-poundingly exciting; it could feel like a trial and a test and go dreadfully wrong. It could be all these things at different moments within the very same relationship, something no child could possibly imagine. But whatever it was, it was a shared process that had a beginning, a middle, and an end, after which one had to go on living and make sense of life without the urgency of desire one had had before the experience. People who say that sex is a simple matter for them are, I think, kidding. Even if one has a gift for it, it still stirs us at the most profound level and goes right to the core of our experience.

On the other hand, eroticism in the larger sense seems like an endless current which, as Salinger said of poetry, flows through all things. When we hear Wagner's *Tristan* or Gershwin's songs, or watch Balanchine's *Bugaku*, we feel it; when I was kissed at that party, I felt it. Eroticism flows through us as an inner sensuality that goes beyond what we do with it; eroticism is our destiny, and we don't need to be having sex at all to be a part of it.

In the end I discovered that the power of sex didn't entirely depend on what "happened." The smallest sexual encounter could carry the charge of the most complete one (every jealous lover knows the truth of this from the other side). Sex has to do with giving and receiving appreciation, with seeing and knowing, being seen and known. It is no coincidence that in the Bible to have intercourse is "to know." Sexual feelings upset our concentration and derail our focus just as much as any panic attack does. Beneath our clothes, beneath our thoughts, we are animals.

Love teaches us to accept the human body. It is the antidote to the horror of it, conveyed by Ernest Becker, in *The Denial of Death,* when he speaks of the realization that we are nothing but a sack of flesh with holes in it. Love for your infant children draws you to them and makes you relish feeding them, holding them, and changing their diapers. Love is the suspension of disgust. It helps us bond with ourselves and with each other. At the same time, it connects with all the other big things; it can't be taken lightly. Love helps us habituate to our arbitrariness.

Up until the age of seventeen I tried to cope with my anxieties without often being in a position to simply avoid the situations I dreaded. Clearly I was not entirely free of social fears, yet if I myself were the center of positive attention or in control of the group, I was able to achieve, it seemed, an uneasy truce between physical distress and the threat of social ostracism, on the one hand, and attention and gratification, on the other. I actually found that being a leader in student government, giving a speech, acting in a play, or later even conducting the music camp orchestra was, terrifying as these activities were, more tolerable than being stuck in the middle of a group. I was willing to trade the pressures of greater responsibility for the freedom of being physically unencumbered and the pleasure of being appreciated. Chairing a meeting or conducting, I could move around. What is more, in these challenging circumstances, my nervousness would at least be more explicable. I still felt wretchedly sick inside, often conducting an entire piece poised to run offstage and throw up, but there was at least the reward of the music itself and the trade-off of personal attention. Nevertheless, this rather agonized, masochistically ritualized way of earning understanding and affection wasn't a secure foundation for a career as a performer. (It strikes me, though, that this type of coping, in which someone becomes in charge of things or a show-off as a way of gaining some control over his own anxiety, must be common. One could imagine that many dictators began their climb to power in such a way.) I also found that by being funny in group situations, I could jump-start my own adaptation to them. I see this mechanism at work in others all the time. I try to be sympathetic to my students when they seem to behave oddly or try to unnerve me in order to get attention. I remind myself that they may be trying to get their bearings instead of fleeing from the classroom, where they are, in a sense, captives. Phobias can lead people to mask their problems in what might seem counterintuitive ways. One way is to become physically ill and be exempted from distressing activities. Another way is to run things yourself, as my father managed to do eventually, so that you can determine your own routines. Such adaptive behaviors can be utterly unconscious.

Throughout college I tensed with apprehension when I rode an elevator or took the subway, and I found classes and all restrictive environments difficult. At times I was dimly aware that my anxiety increased when I was angry about something or suppressing an emotion, even a positive one. In biology class I sat next to a girl I secretly longed for, and sometimes found it hard to breathe. (There is a reason that in the common parlance "heavy breathing" is associated with furtive sexual expression.) I did fly on planes a few times, only gradually—by college's end—reaching a point where I felt I couldn't. Despite the threat of arrest, I attended sit-ins and marches against the Vietnam War. Despite claustrophobia, and to the horror of my parents, I taught a music class at Bridgewater State Prison for a term, barricaded behind a half dozen electronic gates and heavy metal doors at each visit. The feeling of walking under the buzz of fluorescent lights across the barbed-wired courtyard in the twilight, a gray and hopeless stretch of concrete right out of Dostoevsky, stays with me to this day. I wasn't sure at the time what, precisely, my parents worried about in relation to this social work. However, I never did tell them that inmates Chick and Smiley sent me a valentine card.

In my case the onset of true agoraphobia preceded by a year my financial independence from my parents but followed hot on the heels of my (belated) first complete sexual experiences. On the cusp of a weeklong initiation with an old girlfriend who had invited me to stay at her dorm at Vassar College, I embarked on a new relationship with a young Frenchwoman, who, serendipitously, lived in Paris, where I was heading after college. The underlying causality in this love affair could well be questioned, but as so often happens in life, it was no less real for the fact that it rescued each of us in different ways. These were very happy days, and we were tender and comfortable partners. I remember the affectionate simplicity of our weekend afternoons in my sunlit Parisian bed. In retrospect, this was a healthy time. I had successfully finished school and was embarking on an independent life. It's funny how I look back on the period without wistfulness or regret. Perhaps it is actually the truncated, unfinished anguished periods of life that leave one nostalgic and sad. Naturally I had my phobias—and I was lucky enough to be able to travel to France by boat rather than plane—but I was still living expansively. My girlfriend roomed mainly with her mother, but we spent every day together, and many nights.

The following summer, back in the States in between my two years of study in France, things shifted. I started experiencing more anxiety than before. In July I had the bad luck to be stuck in two elevators, I was strangely upset by my girlfriend's anxiety on a bus trip we took together to Montreal (I believe now that her anxiety stirred memories in me of Mary's anguish), I developed a bad case of shingles, and I was composing a piece of music that I knew was dismal, no more than a misshapen collection of Stravinskyan scraps.

At the end of the summer I announced to my parents that my girlfriend would be moving in with me in Paris in the fall, when we returned there together. Something snapped in my mother, and she became almost hysterical. I am still not sure what the central issue was for her, but I do know that I had never really made such a major decision without getting her approval. My father stood up for me, urging her just to accept this new fact, but she was distraught. Was it my mother who was unprepared for this new phase in my life, or was it actually me?

On the boat back to France I had a panic attack almost every day (I was reading Hardy's *Jude the Obscure*, at the time, the darkest novel imaginable and one that concerns incest, marital misery, and a child who murders his siblings and hangs himself), and during the following months the good times were interspersed with incidents of acute anxiety, hypochondria, and confusion. The beautiful streets of Paris suddenly began to look tenebrous and menacing. At first I still rode the metro, even though I would hyperventilate and grow flushed and overheated when it stopped between stations. By late fall I had switched to buses and walking after, as luck would have it, I became stuck in a large metal metro elevator with a group of ten passengers. My stomach and brain registered instantly that the slowing rising cube in which we were encased had come to a premature halt. I asked if anyone there spoke English, and when an elegantly dressed French lady said that she did, I requested that she tell me in English that everything would be all right. She did so in a wonderful French accent, and I still remember the kind expression on her face and the way her lips looked while she was forming the words.

When I received a phone call telling me that my father had suffered a heart attack just before the Christmas holidays, I was told not to come back to see him in case my unexpected visit frightened him. I began to be fearful that I would never make it back to the United States since both boats *and* planes had now become intolerable to me. I feared never seeing my father again.

I panicked at being told for the first time to stay away from home. Is it also possible that without even yet consciously knowing of it, I had somehow instinctively related my father's "rebellion" against my mother to my own? Or that I somehow internally connected the fact that he had stood up for me and my romantic life with his subsequent heart attack? At any rate I became increasingly vulnerable and preoccupied with myself. One time I swallowed a small fish bone at dinner and needed to go to the doctor to be examined and reassured that the bone had indeed eventually gone down where it should have. The tiny scrape it left in my throat preoccupied me for days. Something was "trapped" there, the way I was trapped in Paris and in my psyche. I also had some moments when strange images haunted me. I was disturbed by seeing two dogs locked in intercourse on the street, struggling to come apart. A news program about the separation of the country of Basque (birthplace of Picasso) from Spain also left me weirdly preoccupied. (Merged, then separated, like myself and Mary or like the sex act.)

During this time I composed a brooding theme and variations for piano in a chromatic, atonal idiom far from the airy "French" style I had been exploring. It was still, to be sure, a "student" piece, but it came from inside. My teacher thought that it sounded "like Schoenberg," a composer whom she didn't care for, and said that in her opinion, I was "more direct than that." Nevertheless, she asked me to perform it publicly and praised a passage in which some sad tenths descended in the bass. I remember noting at the time that apparently I had a dark side that was at odds with the sunny face I normally showed people.

During that year in France I began to rein myself in more and more, venturing outside Paris only once—to visit Chartres Cathedral—avoiding subways, trains, and elevators as much as possible, monitoring my physical self and state of mind as if I were somehow an invalid. In spite of this, I took a few driving lessons, which I enjoyed. I recall scurrying around the Place de la Concorde in my little French car, happily navigating the truly maniacal patterns of French drivers. For the most part I clutched myself as if my skin were made of plastic explosives. I identified with my father's illness, fearing that my heart would give out and that the chest pains I felt signaled the proximity of death. I felt suffocated, as if by the very ocean that separated me from the United States and as if only returning to America would permit me to breathe and live. Fortunately, an American doctor counseled me for free and at year's end furnished me with a sedative that made it possible for me to get on a plane back to the States. Even more fortunately, my French girlfriend joined me in New York, and that relationship lasted another five years.

Once I got back to the States, I became much more guarded than I had been. I started avoiding more and more situations and was reluctant to leave the city. I never used the subways or tunnels and even got off buses if they became overcrowded. I felt anxious a great deal of the time, though far less threatened than I had in Europe. My inner calendar was dotted with situations I anticipated with dread. (Next Tuesday: dentist; tenth floor; stairs are locked.) Although my parents helped me pay for visits to a psychiatrist, they quite sensibly told me that in every other respect it was time for me to be financially on my own, and I began a lifelong series of teaching jobs. At a meeting on the twelfth floor of a bank to discuss student loans I was standing, speaking to a bank representative, when the room began to spin and darken. I looked to the windows, as if simply seeing that they could open and imagining air on my face would make me able to breathe. But the windows were sheer glass. (Barlow calls the relief at having an option in an anxious situation the "illusion

of control.") In my dread I remembered the experience of looking down from the upper story of the music room at my school
at the old man lying on the sidewalk fifteen years earlier, when I
was ten. At the bank office, I was amazed that I could remain
upright, while simultaneously imagining myself on the floor
gasping for air. The dizzying moment fused an association between physical and financial disequilibrium, between being unable to open a window and being unable to breathe. That was
when I became acutely aware of whether windows in a building
could be opened or not and began to avoid long, windowless
hallways and modern office buildings.

Fortunately, some summer jobs in the Berkshires helped me
keep circulating. Love, art, and money are great motivators. When
I subsequently married and moved to Vermont, I became almost
as fixed in Vermont as I had been in New York, but I tried to
keep moving enough not to become a recluse. My life evolved
and had many high points, including the fast-moving, often ex-
hilarating days when my children were growing up, but I remained very cautious in the way I lived.

When I started to see a psychiatrist, Dr. Stanley, in the early
1970s, my parents urged me to keep the fact to myself. ("Why
does anyone need to know?") I felt that I had a terrible illness,
whereas my father, who apparently managed without seeing a
doctor, did not. That my mother might be suffering from related
problems never dawned on me. Once when I mentioned her
preoccupation with climatic conditions, she disputed my asser-
tion that she had a "thing" about weather in some detail, for
close to two hours.

I don't pretend to understand what happened when or why,
but I believe that the summer in which I decided to live with my
girlfriend was the moment I went from being someone with
some neurotic quirks—phobias—to being seriously hampered by

agoraphobia. At some points in one's life there is a juncture analogous to the moment when the archduke Francis Ferdinand was
assassinated in Sarejevo in 1914, precipitating the outbreak of
the First World War. The assassination wasn't the true "cause,"
but rather, as one historian puts it, "the *occasion*" for the beginning
of a conflict that had been brewing for decades. So it is in our little lives when fights erupt over who will wash the dishes or
when someone who has been holding it together suddenly can't
anymore. There is a long history beneath such things; they represent a convergence of many strands that happen to meet just at
that point. The evolution of this agoraphobia business was gradual, but it was clinched at the moment I tried to start establishing
my own life. Since then, I now see, I have been dragging a ball
and chain everywhere I go, dragging, in a sense, my childhood
along with me. I have grown up, doing many adult things, while
remaining tethered to the past. This has had, in at least one respect, the same effect that genetic abnormalities, early birth, and
additional psychological imbalances had on Mary: It has slowed
me down.

Would I have become agoraphobic without my mother's
need for me, without her deeply conflicted response to my growth
and independence? Would I have become agoraphobic without
a retarded twin sister who was sent away? Without our remarkable pile-up of family secrets? Was, in fact, any one experience
of crucial importance in determining this aspect of my personality? Such questions are surely unanswerable. My father was
agoraphobic without having had any of the childhood experiences I had. But it is obvious that the many invisible barriers in
the family, in thinking, speaking, and acting, helped reinforce any
existing tendency in me—if it needed reinforcing—*not* to say,
not to do, *not* to explore, and to bury my difficulties inside.
Therefore I arrived at the age of twenty-two not only wary of

life, but deeply ignorant of myself. Mary was rarely mentioned in the family. I was not conscious of the resonances of twinship stirred in me by having a female partner, nor of my terror of being banished by my parents, nor even of my fear of leaving home. Confronted by my mother's sense of alarm at my growing autonomy, instead of rebelling and asserting my rights, I imploded.

In Freud's view, ideal parents will accept the gradual withdrawal entailed by the child's burgeoning independence. Freud could have had my own childhood in mind when he wrote: "The undesirable result of 'spoiling' a small child is to magnify the importance of the danger of losing the object [i.e., the parents] . . . in comparison with every other danger. It therefore encourages the individual to remain in the state of childhood, the period of life which is characterized by motor and psychical helplessness." As a child I had been shielded, protected, and coddled sufficiently for my inner resources to remain slightly less developed than my sense of the perilousness of life. My parents had mixed feelings about my becoming independent and gave me mixed messages about whether I could rely on myself. If one is born with certain sensitivities, as I probably was, that doesn't mean that these sensitivities need to be actively cultivated, as mine were.

An estimable text, entitled *Your Phobia*, written by Manuel D. Zane and Harry Milt, describes what also could be—with slight exaggeration—my own upbringing. That a passage such as this could be almost as accurate about my parents as if the authors had spent the period of my first eighteen years holed up in our family living room taking notes, shows how much uniformity there is in human nature. Zane and Milt note that raising children to be able to face, and bounce back from, the "shocks and losses" of life requires that they be taught that many happenings are simply beyond their control. Sensibly raised children learn that the very best we can do is "to increase the probabilities of safety," but that accidents, tragedies, and difficulties are a part of life and can happen regardless of what we do; they learn that it is self-defeating and absurd to "seek certainty" about what will occur, because there can be no certainty. By contrast, "parents who cannot tolerate uncertainty transmit to their children the attitude that nothing in life is safe, that unless they watch their every step and take absolutely no chances at all, they are likely to suffer some serious and irremediable harm. This sets these children on a course of trying to insure that everything that affects them is safe, that nothing should be done that might possibly harm them. . . . Everything has to follow a definite pattern or a definite formula; any deviation is threatening. Control means certainty and certainty means absolute safety."

Old family habits still dog me. One is that I can express irritation and annoyance or can even be directly critical of people when the environment is more impersonal, but the more intimate the context, the more reticent I become, holding in annoyance even before I know I am doing so. My father was the same way. He could express extraordinary outrage toward Richard Nixon and apparently could blow his stack at work but rarely did so with people close to him. After becoming angry, I always feel as if I have been racked by a terrible storm for which I should apologize. Accustomed as I am to having a "good reason" for whatever I express, rage, when it erupts, is an awful, alien surprise; it feels as if it were coming from someone else.

The price of remaining "rational" about anger and not expressing it as it comes along is that it accumulates inside until it either implodes or explodes, or both. Like my father, I don't seem to know how to express minor annoyance and irritation.

There have been at least a few occassions when I truly erupted: shaking loose a banister in one instance, throwing and breaking plates in another, pounding my fists into a wall in a third, all Darwinian gestures that are remnants of fighting. Memories of these moments later felt out of time, disconnected from the rest of my life.

There is a moment, as I am crossing a bridge, passing under a brief tunnel, or seeing an amazing vista of mountains open up on the road around me, when I feel the thrill of adventure, as if just beneath my fear were desire. Beneath what I cannot do is what I want to do. Beneath all those travel restrictions is that pile of tantalizing maps from the *National Geographic*. Beneath the restrictions are the things I would accomplish if I were less restricted, as well as all the outbursts, the tantrums, the sexual and narcissistic expressions that I have habitually rerouted back to where they came from. Beneath the fear of being suffocated is my muffled self, beneath the fear of vast openness is the fear of being open. Whoever raises you demonstrates his way of expressing or quelling the primary emotions that Damasio writes so brilliantly about, and your first tendency will be to imitate them when you feel these emotions surging through you. I certainly learned a lot from my childhood environment about self-control.

I am always looking for houses on the road, homes, as if I didn't ever get enough of mine. Maybe the houses are really symbols of containment of holding those iron filings in place. I want to stay controlled except where it feels safe not to be: in music. But even when music is playing, even when it's my own, I want to be in an aisle seat.

As I contemplate my agoraphobic tendencies as an adult, it hasn't escaped me that Mary has stayed, to a degree, fixed as she was in one stage of life, remaining forever at the doorway to adulthood, protected from independence. I may even be some-what envious of that protection. I can't help noticing that she, like me, is subject to "attacks," lives within a fixed routine, resists even minute changes from what she expects, is extremely lim-ited in her ability to travel. She is institutionalized, I am out here, "free" and "functioning," yet I have managed to build some invisible walls around myself. I have remained her "twin," finding ways to make my life parallel to hers. In some ways, my parents' intention that I would simply move on in my own way in life has backfired. Regardless of how far away I stay from Mary, her life casts a shadow on mine, as my life shadows hers. Just as I don't feel agoraphobic when I am here at my desk writ-ing, but still am, so forgetting about Mary hasn't changed the truth that we were born together and will always be twins.

In *Emergence,* Temple Grandin vividly described her need for repetition and attachment to routine, as well as her frequent panic attacks, saying that her autonomic nervous system would become unhinged when she went from one setting to another or when-ever she experienced, as she put it, "a lack of sameness in the en-vironment." Perhaps I have a genetic imbalance in my nervous system that overlaps with Mary's in respect to panic. Or perhaps out of guilt or identification I have assumed some of Mary's life restrictions, and this is the very "caramel sauce" I feel has been poured on top of me. At least as of today, there is no MRI in the world that can look into the brain and analyze the neural con-nections to determine which existed in the womb, which were formed at age three, and which were created last month.

When I was in my forties, there was one more major sur-prise in terms of the family history. Right before my father died in 1992, I learned that both my parents had seen psychiatrists for virtually their entire adult lives. The whole time I had been seeking treatment for my problems and they been cautioning me not to mention my treatment to anyone, they had been in treatment themselves. This sense of privacy may have reflected the attitudes of their day, but it also kept me from gaining an accurate perspective on my problems. I doubt that such a scenario would be conceivable today.

There have been rumors from time to time that my mother's psychological upheaval in the thirties was only the first of several. Late in life she acknowledged to her sister that she had had a nervous breakdown years before. I never had the chance to discuss the question with her; the subject was locked in the family trunk of memories along with much else. When, in her eighties, she eventually mentioned her own psychiatric consultations to me, it was to dismiss them as occasions to discuss my father's difficulties with someone.

My parents were very different in their ways of coping with life's tragedies, yet each evaded moments of catharsis, instinctively covering over upsetting truths. "Catharsis" comes from the Greek word meaning "to purge," "to cleanse." Once one has been purged of an emotion, one is perhaps renewed and changed and ready for further changes. My parents kept things fixed. Their relationship to reality was sometimes in itself "agoraphobic," their euphemisms forming detours around places too terrifying to visit, their memories and conversations continually skirting the plain facts, perpetuating the suspicion that a direct look at things could be overwhelming or even annihilating. The family was like a ball of yarn in the center of which all its secrets were tightly bound. It felt as if even the slightest tug on the outer strand could unravel the whole thing.

The map of my mother's world, no less than my father's, was dotted with fixed points of reference, the butcher, the shoe salesman, the pharmacist, people known by name and relied upon. There simply were no other maps.

Our annual trip to visit Mary in Delaware involved being driven over the George Washington Bridge, past the outlets and large companies that line the long, straight, spectacularly banal Route 1 in New Jersey, over the pleasant bridge straddling the Delaware River into Pennsylvania, and eventually into the quiet town where Mary's institution is situated. The ride was terribly difficult for my father, and the sprawling campuslike setting of our destination, with its groups of aging residents, some walking haltingly and bizarrely, some with huge hydrocephalic heads, others hunched over, with brutish, drooping expressions, was a far cry from the comparatively idyllic world of troubled teenagers at Sandpiper in the ocean air of Cape Cod. When these visits were replaced by yearly visits from Mary to see us, they occurred in the summer, in the house my parents rented in Bronxville. (My mother insisted that it could be traumatic for Mary to visit the old apartment in New York.) Mary seemed excited and happy for the most part during lunch, yet also agitated after a little while and eager to get "home" to Delaware. After my father's death my mother did not resume her own visits, and my phobias kept me from making the trip myself. As a result, I maintained the pattern of lunches, and I have seen Mary for precisely two hours each year since that time. I have spent my fifty-seven years holding her at bay, while actually maintaining her inside me.

We are born into life and borne out of it, into the unrecordable, undocumented blankness that can mean whatever we choose it to mean. Hamlet seizes on the pun latent in these two "births" and combines it with the old English word for "region"("bourn") when he speaks of death as

> . . . The undiscovered country, from whose bourn
> No traveller returns . . .

Though any unknown can come to stand for death, it is a false metaphor. Life's unknowns are often knowable; many can be rehearsed or at least imagined. But death is surrounded by an infinite fog on an ocean without end. It is perhaps simplistic to say it, but one can understand death only in terms of its opposite, life. For me, it was always the not returning part of it that made me start up in the dark, suffocating. Yet after my father, who had never even ridden on an airplane, disappeared into that fog, it began to take on other meanings, and I began to dimly see that the not returning part of it is there with us all along, inside us, from the moment we appear into the bewildering new stimuli of the world, even from the moment we start to form out of the fertilized ovum. Now that my mother is gone, it is clearer still. There is only forward motion, and there always was only forward motion. There was never any turning back. The earth itself, once it has fully cooled, will continue to evolve, just as it has never stopped fully evolving. How can we be afraid of that? We can be roused to some deep cosmic dread by this image, perhaps, but who has a mind large enough to truly fear something so beyond anything we can know or will ever know?

"We are born alone and we die alone." For twins, this statement needs to be amended. We are born with company, but we die alone. The early offstage in utero preparations for birth are even now increasingly documented and photographed by microphotography. Who can comprehend what that experience must be like, much less recall it, what it must be like to be forming, to grow eyes, to feel one's fingers separating, to exist without breathing, and slowly awakening to sense? For twins, fraternal or identical, at what point does the mirror become other, do male and female separate, does "one" become "two"?

Mary and I started on the same road. In fact at first we *were* the road. Then we and the road became differentiated, and the road forked, and then we were on two different roads. Who can comprehend such a thing?

Throughout my childhood my parents took pains to emphasize that Mary and I were separate and that fraternal twins are simply brother and sister who happen to be born at the same time. But what is the distinction between the two types of twins in the womb? At what point did I know that Mary's perceptions, her pain, her struggles were distinctly hers and hers alone? And were they, can they ever be? My earliest memory is of sleeping next to Mary, and to this day the sight, smell, and "propinquity" of the female body gives me joy, actually more joy than any touch or affection or any athletic sexual grapplings can ever give.

When I was twelve or thirteen, my piano teacher, Miss Dillon, worked with me on Beethoven's wonderful *Pathétique* sonata. She spoke about Beethoven's "suffering" and reminded me that I knew well what suffering was, although I had yet to encounter the deaths of loved ones, or great physical pain, or great deprivation. She said she knew that I sometimes spent long hours curled up on the floor of my bathroom with a stomachache. I suppose my mother must have worried openly to her about this, despite her ambivalence about Miss Dillon's possessive and nurturing interest in me, her delightfully frank and extroverted manner. My suffering may not have been earthshaking, but like my first awkward creative efforts, it did deserve respect, simply because it was mine. Miss Dillon had it right. Like the music of Tchaikovsky's *Swan Lake,* her words seemed to give me permission to be as old as I was.

Everyone has a story. In the grand scheme of things, my life contains a bare minimum of external pressures. By any objective measure, mine was a fortunate childhood. Like all childhoods, it had its wrinkles and bumps, which, in tandem with my inborn topography, left marks on the map of my current behavior. It makes sense that agoraphobia struck me in full force in early adulthood. In a way I had been raised to feel that the world was a kind of Pandora's box that was simply too frightening to ever fully open. As an adult I found a way to open it a bit, while sitting on top of it too.

My mother may have found my transition to adulthood terrifying, but in the end there was also a gradual letting go on her part until at the point that I had children myself, she warmly embraced the stage of life we all had arrived at. She loved being with her grandchildren and showered upon them the kindness and playful delight she had always shown young people. After my father's death she became more and more accepting of changes. Eventually she displayed an astounding imperviousness to her own ailments and impairments. She remained uninterested in the medical details but was actually a stoical realist about aging.

As I write this, my mother has only just died, at the age of ninety-nine. In her last few years her mind was in shadow. She lost the ability to speak, except occasionally to outline a few words with her mouth, and she could not walk or take care of herself in any way. Yet up until close to the end one sensed that her attention was still directed outward, as it always had been, and that in some region, words spoken to her registered and had meaning. One felt that she was still there, inside.

Bafflingly, she now exists in my memory in all the phases of her life that I knew. I can easily picture her as she was fifty years ago, making me a beautiful alligator costume for Halloween, and

I can picture her as she was six years ago, still able to follow the presidential election campaign in minute detail.

I also see her as she was a year ago, opening her eyes, taking her time to register who I am, remaining courteously formal until she is no longer in doubt. She brightens by degrees. When she sees it is me, her hazel brown eyes sparkle, and she beams. The shrewdness and canniness that marked her up until so recently have etched habits into her facial expressions, but her tensions and her impulse to control things are gone. Speechless, a joy in communication remains; her kindness remains. Her eyes are still romantic, beautiful, and expressive. She is tiny, yet astoundingly strong.

I didn't always appreciate how formidable she was. I believe that while my father was alive, she couldn't help resisting almost anything that might further destabilize her marriage; this included anything she might have done to assert her own independence and creativity. She had an unshakable command of grammar and spelling and a phenomenal memory for political details. She convinced a number of friends to oppose the Vietnam War through the sheer volume of information she was able to bring to bear on her arguments. Yet she could also deliberately mask the force of her mind. Not coincidentally, she also resisted much of what my brother and I did to assert our independence.

But once my father was not there, and we were now her "men," she directed toward us the optimistic and progressive personality that our father had relied upon throughout their marriage. This transformed my relationship with her, making it delightful and even liberating to be with her. She was proud of my brother and me not only for what we did but for what we were trying to do. As much as she delighted in his successes as an actor, she admired my brother even more for his writing and for his human qualities—his brilliance, courage, and goodness. She adored his friends from the world of avant-garde theater, and she helped me pay for some of my recordings, expressing her excitement that I wrote music that was "of my time." In her last years she seemed to exude a kind of cheerful faith in the possibilities of the future.

Chapter Twelve

Alone/Not Alone

If we cannot see things clearly we will at least see clearly where the obscurities are.
—SIGMUND FREUD

I would like to attend the ceremony if I were able to. But unfortunately I'm mentally ill with agoraphobia. I'm unable to be in crowds and I can't bear to be looked at.
—ELFRIEDE JELINEK, ON NOT ATTENDING THE CEREMONY IN STOCKHOLM AWARDING HER THE 2004 NOBEL PRIZE IN LITERATURE

. . . The best way out is always through.
—ROBERT FROST

It was something of a shock to be in a roomful of phobia sufferers at New York's Roosevelt Hospital. Back then, in the late seventies, such support groups, modeled on addiction programs, group therapy, and political cells, were a new idea. My group was predominantly female, with the exception of a detective with a heights phobia. One of the therapists was a recovered agoraphobic and the other was an avowedly anxious psychiatrist. It was the first time I had heard of the notion of coping with anxiety or of the idea that some people simply have to face being more anxious than others. The other two great revelations were that phobias came in so many different shapes and sizes and that there were apparently enough serious phobics in the world to form a nation with the population of India.

The program included group discussions, relaxation exercises, working through a handbook, individual sessions with a trained helper who would accompany one into dreaded situations, and nervous outings with fellow sufferers. With fellow phobic Denise, I went to the sixth floor of a crowded Bloomingdale's and ventured deep into Central Park, standing in a field. Wide spaces bothered her even more than they did me, and coaching her breathing was something like being in Lamaze class. My "aide" drove me across the Fifty-ninth Street Bridge while I narrated the level of my anxiety and symptoms; she stood next to me in hushed elevators ascending to the top floor and down, as normal people got on and off, living their lives. The weekly groups involved information sessions, patient progress reports, and sometimes discussions of people's marriages or interpersonal tensions. Afterward I would share a taxi with Clara, a sex therapist who told me about penile implants and other things I had never heard of before.

The group treatment was my psychiatrist Dr. Stanley's idea and its initiation was the first time I recognized that a lifetime of talking and remembering would not undo my "phobia" problem. It must sound remarkably naïve, but until the first day of the Roosevelt clinic, I had assumed that phobias, or gambling, alcoholism, violent behavior, or extreme shyness, resulted from the way your childhood had gone and were a kind of curse that could be lifted if you could talk your way to the magic spell. If you recalled the pertinent memory or offending influence, a beautiful angel with a golden key would suddenly descend, like the duck with a hundred-dollar bill in its beak on the Groucho Marx show, and unlock your chains.

Dr. Stanley was not my first psychiatrist. Almost fifteen years earlier as a college freshman I had sought the help of a benevolent aging professor of psychology who happened to be a friend of a friend and also someone I ran into occasionally at concerts. These facts made me trust him enough to ask for a consultation, even though his office was on the twelfth floor of the Psychology Center. At the time I had only recently confessed to my mother that I was often unbearably anxious. The professor saw me weekly for free for two months before referring me to a younger psychiatrist whose dry, squeamish manner—which managed to communicate both distaste and a deep pessimism about life— completely alienated me. I dropped the psychological approach for the rest of my college years. The professor had favored a technique called deconditioning, which bordered on hypnosis. He had me stare at a small model of the Eiffel Tower that glinted in the light of a desk lamp, while he talked me through states of progressive relaxation. Then he would have me imagine being in the subway, or in an elevator, or on a plane.

In retrospect the little Eiffel Tower came to seem like a sign of some kind, a harbinger of the free, sunny days I would enjoy in Paris after graduation. Of course those sunny days, lucky and wonderful as they were, became progressively clouded by my internal problems, until the clouds came close to overwhelming me. At that point, fearing that I would be unable to return home, I again sought psychological help, at the Paris "American Center," and, once back in New York, entered "therapy" seriously at a free clinic with a psychologist intern, Dr. Wiessen. Since I was considered articulate, Dr. Wiessen had me designated the subject of a classroom presentation on phobias. I was put up onstage under lights in a darkened auditorium, and psychology students my own age and younger asked me questions about how it felt to be phobic. The experience was humiliating and unnerving.

After two years Dr. Wiessen left New York, and I sought another referral through my medical doctor. Following an interim clinical evaluation I was referred to the serious, likable, and highly intelligent Dr. Stanley, a man who revealed enough of his own artistic tastes and lifestyle to make me feel that we inhabited the same world and that I was not a freak. While our sessions helped me, the phobias remained. I occasionally tried medications in order to undertake this or that challenge or simply to endure some experiences better, but they left me feeling troubled, flat, and empty, as if the experience had happened to someone else.

My participation in the Roosevelt group clinic was far from a complete loss. It gave me a dawning understanding of the problem and some useful coping techniques, enough to make moving out of New York and learning to drive possible. A subsequent series of sessions at the Center for Stress and Anxiety Disorders ten years later was also valuable. Three years ago I resumed a similar form of treatment. Although I am still struggling and can't predict how much better I will get, the treatment programs I attended have helped me expand my routine and to function within it with less anxiety. I have also overcome difficulties I had never before noticed having.

The treatment approach is based on the premise that in order to get over serious phobias, one needs to start building up a new history of experiences with the phobic situations/triggers, experiences in which one endures them, copes better with them, or even eventually is not terribly disturbed by them. Imagine what it does to your brain and to your thought patterns when you spend years systematically avoiding something, reinforcing its power as an object of dread so terrible that it can kill you. A new experience in which you practice enduring what you once refused to do is a step toward revising your history in the situation, creating instead the kind of normal ambivalence we all have about things that are unpleasant but that we have learned to tolerate.

Deconstructing the phobic process involves not only dismantling the physiology of anxiety but also analyzing the assumptions and split-second habits of mind that constitute its cognitive side. The cognitive aspect of a phobia has four basic components: (1) the way we interpret what is happening in the moment of phobic response; (2) the thoughts and associations that accompany this experience; (3) the unconscious emotions and memories stirred by it; and (4) the underlying function of phobias in our life, the reason we may have resorted to "using" phobias to avoid things (secondary gain). Cognitive/behavioral therapy helps one dismantle the strands of so-called catastrophic thinking that help fuel the arousal of the body in fear. It deconstructs the various symptoms of anxiety through explanation and exercises designed to initiate each one in turn and demystify it. One studies what anxiety is, learns many strategies for managing it, and works on facing the phobic object with new thinking and relaxation techniques.

The phobic process itself can take on personal meanings. Many people report feeling as if they were going insane when in a panic state. This sense of mental turmoil had a particular meaning for me. Along with it came memories of the anguish that so overwhelmed Mary when she was upset. It took me years to recognize that the experience of derealization and depersonalization reminded me of her, or to relate my panic to Mary's own desperate childhood outbursts, since I learned neither to incorporate Mary into my life nor to have a realistic sense of our separateness.

Of course as a first step I needed to learn that there was a psychological dimension to panic for everyone. Then, when faced with panic, I actually began to speak to myself out loud, to tell myself that I was still there, that I hadn't come apart, that I still had Mary in my life, but that I wasn't becoming her. As a result, I felt at least a dawning awareness, in my fifties, that it might be possible for me to come to terms with some of the experiences I had avoided. I believe that if I had that dawning awareness at all, it was due as much to the investigations I did in conventional therapy as to the practical training I received from the cognitive/behavioral therapy. Eventually these together spurred me to visit Mary on her home ground.

My first experience at the Roosevelt clinic more than twenty-five years ago was significant to me in a deeper way than as a source of information or demonstration of the healing powers of practice. As with all conditions that are outside the ordinary, being seriously phobic can engender enormous shame. In addition to whatever social phobias a person may have, severe phobias can bring with them the fear of discovery and of becoming an outcast. Shame begins inside, with being afraid to admit, even to oneself, that one is in some respects hampered. This adds to the claustrophobia of living in an artificially restricted way, the claustrophobia of keeping one's condition trapped inside oneself. This shame mitigates not only against change, since even a small degree of change presupposes the admission of a problem, not only against becoming informed, since receiving information requires asking for it, but also in the end against hope.

The almost universal expression of shame is the downward cast of the head, the averted gaze. How can one avert one's gaze, on the one hand, and regard people frankly, on the other? In some sense, being ashamed of one aspect of oneself holds the rest of the personality hostage. Being ashamed alters one's stance toward the world. Admitting that one is not well actually liberates all that is healthy. My experience at the Roosevelt clinic did not relieve my shame, but it at least taught me that I was one of many with such problems. It placed me in a community of fellow sufferers where shame could be forgotten. It paved the way for me to acknowledge a side of my life that I preferred to pretend wasn't there.

It was during the same period that I started to confront my phobias at the clinic that I first learned of my father's other household and had my first of several long conversations with him about it. From the moment I brought the subject up he seemed relieved—relieved to talk about it and relieved that I didn't reproach him. Although his other relationship had come as a complete surprise to me—I had never consciously thought that anything about his routine required explanation—I felt this relief too. While I saw my parents as a loving couple, I had never actually viewed them as an indissoluble unit, like a salt and pepper shaker. I took pleasure in their individuality. Just as I had always loved seeing the unadorned face of my mother, without makeup, so I deeply enjoyed seeing the more complete, unencumbered father I discovered in these talks with him.

His story was one I could at least partially identify with, yet some aspects of what he said did not seem like the whole truth. For example, he said that he would have discussed things openly with my brother and me were it not for my mother's inability to handle it. I could see that he was in fact completely comfortable discussing it with me. Yet I was inclined to think that the policy of secrecy served the interests of both my parents. I saw my father as maintaining an unorthodox equilibrium—between different sides of himself, between different types of love, even between different ways of living—that, while often painful and strained, was his way of coping with life. (With characteristic understatement he described the complex duality of his arrangements as "not recommended.") A greater openness across the board would have transformed, or ended, our family life and, at the very least, would have altered his carefully compartmentalized routine. By virtue of this compartmentalization his two relationships could be different, yet each could be experienced as complete in itself.

At the same time, I was angered to realize that neither of my parents had ever worried that their silence on the topic, which after all couldn't go on forever, might have had its own deleterious effect on my brother and me. Yet at what point does a marital crisis become a "way of life," suitable for open discussion?

Psychologist Ron Cohen, who has had a lifelong interest in the subject of silence, talks about how the inability to discuss a taboo subject can represent a kind of blockage akin to a phobia. "We think of silence as an absence of talk, as somehow simply an empty space. In actuality it can mean different things, and it can truly have solidity," he told me. "It can be built into the very structure of life without anyone being able to see it—in a family, in an institution, in a country. This happened in families in relation to the Holocaust, for example, where people played exquisitely detailed games in their families to avoid speaking about the elephant that was right there in the room."

I mentioned the obvious parallels with families in which there is alcoholism or incest.

"That's right," said Ron. "Silence can take the form of being afraid to bring something up, afraid to say something. In this form it is like a phobia, an obstruction, an emblem for a fear that is not necessarily even understood. Sometimes we think: 'I don't know why I can't bring myself to say this.' As with phobias, people go through all kinds of diversionary tactics in order to avoid coming out with a direct statement."

The concept of diversionary tactics led me to mention the connection one could make between my being agoraphobic and having had all these family secrets, like roads one couldn't go down. Conversationally, imaginatively, I had to take detours around unpleasant facts. "When it comes to delving into taboo subject matter or bringing up a painful subject," I said to Ron, "we even have the colloquial expression: 'Don't *go* there.'"

Ron nodded vigorously. "Right you are," he said. "We say, 'Don't go there,'" at which point we lapsed into another kind of silence, as perhaps we each contemplated some of the inner places to which we couldn't "go."

In terms of the elephant in our family living room involving my father's double life (one elephant of several), more open discussion certainly didn't cure my travel phobias. But it did free up a spring of feeling thwarted at the source by lies and obfuscation. When one's perceptions are not given credence or one is being deceived, one doesn't feel properly loved. My parents had kept me from knowing an important part of their history and in the process warped my relationships with them. Thankfully, in the last years of my father's life and then in the final years of my mother's, many of the old barriers were removed.

I had always felt connected to my father's passionate side. I have no doubt that it was the directness of his emotional expression at the piano that turned me into a musician. While his own warmth and concern always communicated themselves through his restrained nature—he was one of the most communicative people I have ever met—the moments when he truly let his guard down were enormously reassuring. His temperamental balance couldn't be imitated. Neither my brother nor I could actually live our lives in the way he did. As growing men we soaked up with eagerness the moments when he "cut loose," to use his own words. Such instances often occurred in precisely those situations that he anticipated with anxiety. Seeing him, as I once did, run across the floor of an airport lobby because there was a rumor that the Beatles were getting off a plane at that very moment or seeing him dance with a shapely young woman at an all-night diner in Vermont or relish a performance of one of my brother's plays in a cramped theater in lower Manhattan—surely a nervous-making adventure for him—confirmed me in my own possibilities. Once, a few hours after a hernia operation in the late 1960s, my father talked to me from his hospital bed with the sodium pentathol still flowing through him. Speaking in a strong voice, rich with an almost drunken pleasure, he lovingly introduced me to the nurse attending him, saying, "This is my son." He seemed so unburdened and so connected to life lying there in his hospital pajamas, still semi-anesthetized. He seemed more than usually able to acknowledge his feelings and his connections. Under sodium pentathol he became the man who played the piano and the ruddy-faced man I had seen at the office. I have to admit that I almost felt a sense of letdown when the anesthesia wore off. Such moments were welcome confirmations of the fullness with which the life force flowed through him. For the same reason, although I might have viewed the subject as a threat to my own world, I in fact felt satisfaction and a sense of fulfillment during the conversations I had with him about his romantic life.

In my search to understand the phobia problem better I attended a session of Fly Without Fear at La Guardia Airport last year. I went not because I intended to get back on a plane in the near future but to make contact with the feeling of hope I knew I would find there. I was uncomfortable with the daytime drive from Vermont to New York this required. (I naturally packed the doughnuts I carry with me on every trip like a religious talisman.) I had to fight the urge not to continue the drive several times along the way. Upon arriving in Manhattan four hours later, I had to resist the desire to turn around before taking the Triborough Bridge to the airport. And once at the airport, when

I became hopelessly confused by the various ramps and signs, I had to fight the urge, more than once, to leave right then and there.

I could pretend that I disgraced myself by entering the third-floor conference room late and out of breath or that I was mercilessly mocked when I took my place in the available front row seat, but that would not be true. The room was too full of apprehensive fellow phobics for my late entrance to be noteworthy.

As I collected myself in my chair, I could feel the surface tension in the audience perceptibly vibrating. As Carol Cott Gross, a lifelong claustrophobic and the indefatigable director of Fly Without Fear, addressed and cajoled her members, anxiety was etched on their faces. A wave of fellow feeling surged over me, mixing with my own inner tensions. The realization that had come to me when I first attended the Roosevelt sessions returned. It was the observation, so obvious I always seem to forget it, that as alone as we all are with our sensations and experiences, our struggles and our flaws, our lives and our deaths, we are also linked to one another from the moment of conception to death. We may be geared to view life from a single perspective—the solitary "I" that experiences life and feels pain—but at a subterranean level we are part of larger patterns in every domain that we are simply too self-centered, to observe. We are each unique yet, in most basic respects, completely unoriginal.

Sitting with my fellow phobics in Fly Without Fear I discerned two basic types of people: those whose anxiety was somewhat visible and those who seemed to have a tendency—one I share—to appear relatively comfortable even while suffering acutely. But all belonged to the millions who experience extraordinary pain negotiating the seemingly painless. Carol did not speak of overcoming her own claustrophobia, only of overcoming some of the restrictions she had placed on herself as a result of it. "This is like a blood type," I thought. "We are people with our dials set a certain way. It is as if we all descended from the mating of two anxious lovers on the isle of Phobos, the land of the nervous, long ago. This phobic reaction is just built in, our particular fault line, the place where we tend to erupt in reaction to the crisis of being."

This type of revelation comes to all those who discover that their private shame is shared by a sizable segment of the population, and is a phenomenon with a name and well-documented characteristics.

"How easy it is to get tied up in knots," I was thinking, as Carol spoke. "And then how very long it takes to patiently untie each knot separately, hoping one day to recover that original ball of string. . . ."

Carol talked about the terrors of the current world, including terrorism in Israel and London, two places where members had recently flown. She spoke about the irony that they had dreaded the flights more than the realistic dangers of the trips themselves. She talked about the superstition inherent in phobia, how the members assume the worst about their own flights yet have confidence when family or friends fly. She talked about how phobics don't like to relinquish control. "We are Type A personalities," she was saying. "Many phobics don't like to take medication because they fear the loss of control. We are vigilant. God forbid there might be an emergency and then we might actually be relaxed! We have to learn to hand over control to the pilot of the plane. We need to meet the pilot and mentally hand over the controls to him. We cannot fly the plane. He can. He knows what he is doing." I thought of my dear mother and our closely monitored cab rides down Fifth Avenue and across the park at Sixty-fifth Street.

Carol herself is a fighter. After lying in bed with a back injury, she decided not to let her phobias restrict her traveling. She routinely flies to Europe. She had just returned from Berlin. "But if it were up to me," she was saying, "I would still stay at the same hotel every single time because it is familiar to me. That's because I am a phobic." Yes, I thought, in our childhood, the unquestioned assumption behind virtually any action was that doing things *the same way as last time* was good.

Carol expanded on the topic of habituation. "If we all sat on the plane in the hangar a bit every day for a month," she said, "I guarantee you that much of your fear would disappear, even if we never took off, because you would become *used to the environment*." This thought reminded me of a few moments that I had in fact experienced: walking down the "empty" road, for instance, or driving to Montreal, when suddenly I would relax and the view would suddenly be simply what happened to be there, where my need to worry about where exactly I was simply dissolved. Carol congratulated everyone for attending the session, pointing out that there were many who considered themselves members and had even often mailed in their admission fees, who had never yet made it to a meeting.

A marvelous woman, a painter who was a veteran of five years of attending Fly Without Fear, spoke of a flight in which she had had a panic attack. "It was fine," she said. "It happened, and then . . ."

"You ran out of adrenaline" said Carol. "How long does a panic attack last? Twelve minutes, maybe up to twenty."

"Yes, it subsided. Afterward I felt good," added the speaker, "because if you are doing the thing you want to do, you experience a feeling of accomplishment and optimism when you face into the panic, and just move forward." And I thought: "It is not the bridge, or the tunnel, or the flight, but your body's and mind's reaction, always the same, that you need to learn to cope with."

As we descended the stairs to the hangar, I virtually clung to Carol, my breaths becoming short as we passed through several long, windowless hallways, way past the point where I would know how to retrace my steps. It was a bit like being backstage at one of the large theaters at which I used to work as a pianist in New York. There was the same sense of being behind the scenes, in a work environment full of tools, electrical cables, and props that the audience never sees. I tried to focus on that, but I felt disoriented and unglued. We passed a glamorous female flight attendant heading toward her "dressing room" in street clothes. "Visiting?" she asked.

"Fear of flying," answered a member.

"Oh," she said, smiling. "I'm not afraid."

The hangar opened out to the night like a gigantic garage with its door raised. Through it came a summer breeze and glimpses of a few lights twinkling far off. We boarded a plane that was being inspected and tuned up inside the hangar. Occasionally the rumble of a nearby departure shook the space. There were enough of us to fill a large portion of the plane. Some of the anxiety of the meeting room yielded to surprise and interest. I wouldn't call it a carnival atmosphere, but there was a lifting out of self that came from actually being there, in a place you wished not to be, but would need to be if you wanted to see the world. Carol explained that the heat of the plane exacerbated claustrophobia. When the "air" was turned on, it did have a relaxing effect. I thought of countries I most wanted to visit: France again, of course . . . Austria to visit Vienna, where Mozart and Beethoven and Schubert and Schoenberg had lived . . . England . . . Japan, home of composer Toru Takemitsu, of filmmakers Yasujiro Ozu and Akira Kurosawa, of writers Junichiro Tanizaki and Banana Yoshimoto. . . . The tension in my legs ebbed and flowed. Bob, the plane's engineer, made his way up the center of the plane with the expression of a man for whom planes were close to everything. Like the captain and crew of the ship I took to Europe, for whom land life had become alien, Bob, I imagined, was someone for whom not knowing every aspect of the world of planes would be close to unimaginable. He explained that the plane was in the hangar for a routine inspection. He offered to show us the cockpit, and I took him up on it. It was a tiny, cramped space like a racing car with seats for two, bedecked with handsome, brightly lit dials.

The plane door remained open. Soon we descended and returned to the parking lot and our cars. Like the technique my friend P. had tried with moths, this was a rare opportunity to touch a piece of reality that one had held at bay. I was impressed by how brave the members of the group were.

Afterward I spoke with a painter who told me about her phobias, about her love of travel and foreign languages.

"Fortunately," she said, "I have a therapist who is action-oriented and practical. He had me practice taking elevators. I have begun to outgrow some of my phobias, such as those of subways and bridges. He told me that avoidance makes the fear stronger. He taught me—I know this sounds simplistic, but it actually works—'Don't think your way into right action; act your way into right thinking.' I am a very moody person, and I am very affected by my surroundings, in a good sense. When I am uncomfortable, I put myself in a new circumstance, and I feel changed. When I was in Asia, I was euphoric. If I tried to simply 'think' my way into right action, I wouldn't do anything."

Looking at the map, one wouldn't imagine that the trip to Mary's institution would be all that difficult, but the closer I got to her, the more obstacles there seemed to be. I was tremendously eager to see her, in her own place, and to meet with her doctors there, but often it seemed, at various points along the way, simply undoable. Although the trip would have been difficult even if the goal was simply a concert or an important occasion, there was clearly more in the way than even "phobia."

I drove halfway there two years ago but made it only as far as the border of New Jersey. Before that trip I hardly slept, dreaming fitfully of my son, then fifteen, who had recently grown to be six feet tall. In my dream his younger self stood proudly next to his new self, looking up. There were two of him: one a boy, the other a grown man.

The next morning I was tired from lack of sleep and grew exhausted from the tension. When I reached the entrance to a highway I hadn't expected, I had been on the road for six hours, and I balked. I turned around and tried another way. Stalemate. I again turned around, parked, gathered my forces, tried again. I was frozen in place, like a cornered animal. I returned sadly to Vermont.

Two weeks ago I studied the map again and found an alternative route. I tried again and made it past the "barrier," far enough to feel more confident about the trip. But as soon as I had made it past that point, I felt a new kind of dread. The goal again receded, a dark conundrum, part external, part internal.

Last week I again made the attempt. Far from being easier than expected, it was in fact harder. I felt like the little dung beetle in the insect documentary *Microcosmos,* pushing a dung ball no bigger than a child's marble up a steep incline, gathering all its energies for the tiny triumph of successfully reaching the top.

Here I was, a lucky person with no physical handicap, lifting the weight of an ordinary day as if it were a boulder five times my size.

I woke nauseated and dizzy on the morning of the trip. My first waking thought was: "I can't possibly go." It took a strong cup of coffee to stimulate the perception that I was probably more anxious than ill and that even if I was sick, I should still go. Before leaving, I impulsively did all my laundry and then became preoccupied with whether or not I should leave my socks paired or unpaired until I returned. (I left them unpaired.) I got into the car in a state of befuddlement and jangled nerves.

I had decided to break the trip in half. I reserved a room in a motel somewhat beyond the achieved goal of the previous week. This would mean I would have, at most, only a three-hour drive ahead of me, as the final leg of the journey, the following morning. Along the road I felt a frequent impulse, coming with the force of the cargo in the hold of a ship lurching to the opposite side of the boat, to turn around. I encountered several confusing moments in the route and had to retrace my steps several times. As usual this was accompanied by a sense of the grotesque. "This is New Jersey, for God's sake," I thought, "not an Arctic crossing." At one point in the trip, retracing my steps, I came to a crossroads and stopped in the middle of it in bewilderment, just as a fire engine barreled by at eighty miles per hour, narrowly missing me. The difference between good luck and bad luck is sometimes measured by an inch. Phobia-Fear coursed through me. I parked on the side of the road to let the tempo of my heart slacken. I checked the map. I waited ten minutes for my eyes to retrieve their focus. I saw my mistake on the map. I resumed.

From time to time I tried a trick I learned at the anxiety clinic. Tension begets tense behavior. Relaxed behavior aids relaxation. By deliberately gripping the steering wheel lightly, I fooled myself into feeling more relaxed.

From the cross-hatchings of memory sprang the heat of my father's overcoated presence in the old car trips down Route 1; I sensed his leaden mood as he went over manuscripts line by line, sometimes raising his bespectacled eyes, pen in hand, to ponder sifting out a word or phrase. I thought of riding a train with my mother from Bronxville into Manhattan to see a French movie starring Leslie Caron, on a bright summer day when I was eight, of the contrast between the summer sunlight and the darkened theater, of something inexpressibly sad in my mother's cheerfulness and in its being just us two.

Reaching the motel quite drained, I had an unexpected mental image, like a waking dream. I saw Mary before me, and I slapped her. "How could you put me through this?" I was yelling. "How could you?" In my imagination she burst into tears, baffled, and said my name, and said, "What are you doing, Allen? That's not nice, Allen," and I cried, and she cried. . . .

I had never imagined or experienced such a moment, nor had I ever had such an unbidden mental image. It seemed like an outcry, as if my anguish about reaching her were mixed up with my anguish that she was so hard to understand, as if our fates were mixed up together (as they are), as if I could never forgive her for making believe that she couldn't express herself more normally.

Weirdly there was a show on television in which an agoraphobic artist was accused of a crime. He hadn't left his apartment in a few years. The beautiful policewoman was convinced of his innocence only when he was shot by the real perpetrator. After being rushed from his apartment to the hospital, he recovered from the shooting and, amazed to be no longer trapped in his apartment, began to face his agoraphobia. The show ended as he walked in the park arm in arm with the policewoman.

Gradually I dozed off.

I awakened at 3:30 A.M. in a sweaty panic, with my heart and breathing in full throttle, and a sense of in extremis loneliness, having dreamed continuously, it seemed, of being reproached. In my dreams I was trying to be reconciled with those I had hurt. I dreamed of my children, of a colleague I hadn't seen for years with whom I had once fought; I dreamed of my mother. There were tears, there were things that had come apart, coming together, but not quite. In my dreams no one would look at me. I now lay in bed burning up and trembling at the same time. I thought of the town asleep around me, the strangers, the dead silence, the roads leading confusingly this way and that, through deserted farmlands with their yellow fields lying in shadow, of endless miles of deserted train tracks, and of all the dark homes with people asleep in them, people who didn't know me and who would probably reach for a shotgun if I knocked on their door in the middle of the night and begged them for help. I wondered what would happen if the motel personnel found me dead in the morning. Would my identity cards make a trail to people who cared about me? I lay that way for an hour and a half, trying to remember how to breathe. Eventually I returned to my dreams.

Things looked better at 7:30 A.M. I tried to ride the moment of optimism that sometimes comes with waking. I tried to ride on the current of what is normal. My pushing paid off.

Three hours later I sat with Mary, visiting her alone for the first time ever, in a place where I had not been for twenty-seven years. There was Mary. It is not easy to describe something so entirely ordinary and also slightly overwhelming. Psychologists call the bonding of early relationships imprinting. The formative people in your life are in your cells. I experienced Mary's presence with an indefinable emotion, essential, yet as colorless as water. Mary seemed so pleased to see me. She took my hand with a strong grip and showed me her room and walked around with me just as I remembered from childhood. She offered me the top of her head to kiss, just as my father used to do. She shied away from a firm hug, though, an averting I now understood from Temple Grandin's writings.

For Mary, time never seems to pass. Whether or not I am bald, or have a beard, or my hair has turned gray, the connection to me is simply "now." For me time collapses when I see her; everything seems to make sense. Being with her locates the source of a strange feeling I carry around with me everywhere. I wouldn't be myself without her. Yet I can never know her the way one normally "knows"—or imagines one does—other people.

I felt an overwhelming sense of my parents' and brother's presence when I was with Mary, a sense of my parents' DNA in the room, of the poignancy of her continuing so much that was theirs even after their deaths, but I also felt that their particular sorrow, their heaviness, was not my own. For me there was a lightness in being with Mary, a lifting of pretense. I have never known a world without Mary. To be with her was to touch something sad, confusing, and even shocking and yet to feel well.

When I met with Dr. Trombley, Mary's psychiatrist, I heard a new account of her diagnosis. In a sense it was a return to the original one, shorn of the violence inherent in the notion of birth trauma.

"It seems to me that Mary is a classic autistic," he said. "She has certain characteristics that show up only with autism. For example, delayed echolalia, when people repeat phrases verbatim from previously heard conversations or movies or video games and fit them into the conversations they are having.

Temper outbursts in autistic kids are not uncommon because they have a need to have the world conform to their demands. Also, they are bothered by certain touches and noises and feel easily overwhelmed by stimuli the rest of us take in stride. When we see autistic kids not tolerating changes and noises, we know that they are not processing the world as we are. If you bring them to certain places, a shopping mall, say, they cannot cope.

"Some autistics develop bipolar disorder in later life. A small percentage develop psychotic disorder in addition to autism. Mary started having severe psychotic episodes in the early 1970s, which included hallucinations, erratic behavior, and self-mutilation. With verbal people like Mary, you can tell when they are responding to something that is not present in the room. That is when she was diagnosed as having schizo-affective disorder. This means that she is having mood swings accompanied by schizophrenic symptoms. This is when she was put on medication.

"In the fifties autism was regarded as stemming from upbringing, the old 'refrigerator mom' idea. Today it is almost universally regarded as the result of genetic defects, a matter of flaws in the way the genes have directed the brain to form, and the neurons in the brain to fire and how quickly to connect. About one-third of autistics have a normal or above normal IQ. But roughly two-thirds of autistics are mentally retarded. However, many of them have extraordinary abilities that exceed the normal. So the fact that you were premature and in incubators is probably not the source of the problem at all. It is highly unlikely that what happened to Mary occurred at birth or after birth. Her autism was surely determined prebirth, in utero."

I asked him if there was a connection between the rest of our family's need for routine and Mary's powerful need for order and complete consistency, her anguish when certain things—holidays, food, her living quarters—are not exactly as she expects them to be.

"It is hard to say," he answered. "You do find certain patterns in families of autistics. A pattern of shyness, for example. It is certainly possible that there are shared family influences. At the same time it is possible that when Mary got four of a certain flawed gene, you got two. In some ways you are just sister and brother. But even as fraternal twins, sharing fifty percent of your DNA, as you would with any sibling, you are still closer to each other than to any other people on earth, closer than a brother and sister born two years apart, for instance. New studies of the human genome are beginning to shed light on some significant ways in which infants are affected by the biochemical environment in the womb. Apart from your genetic connection, you and Mary shared this formative environment at the same exact moment. Whatever your mother experienced during pregnancy affected you equally."

I needed nothing more from this small trip than to see Mary, but in the end I also derived from it a much deeper understanding of how each of us had come to be, how and why we differed, and what it meant that we were twins. I had made an important step toward reconnecting wih her. I had also made a step toward reconnecting with the fundamental truths of my life and toward finding the source of the "piercing scream" I seem always to hear when there is nothing around me to shield me from it.

Epilogue

I'm not afraid of death. I just don't want to be there when it happens.
—WOODY ALLEN

Someday, and scientists have apparently calculated approximately when, the process of the Earth's creation will be reversed. The sun's power will diminish, the Earth's core will cool, and not only will we and our most distant descendants be gone, but even the planet itself will revert to being inhospitable to life. Yet it is rare to encounter someone with a phobia of the death of the sun. Perhaps there are those who panic at the sight of the map of the world as it may have looked in the Cambrian period, five hundred million years ago, when the continents were bunched up in the lower latitudes of the globe, dormant, misshapen, un-recognizable, wrong. But such a reaction is exceptional. It is also a rare person who feels panicky at the mention of ancient times, historical periods when only his most distant ancestors walked the earth.

We tend to be phobic about the things we might actually confront in the future, things within our frame of reference. It is not the idea of a Martian that disturbs us; it is the idea of a Martian who knocks on our door.

Yet the sense of our cosmic irrelevance, the sense of our not being necessary, lies in wait for us in our psyches, ready to spring up unexpectedly. In *Speak Memory* Vladimir Nabokov, referring to himself in the third person, writes of being overcome with alarm seeing photographs of his parents and his childhood home taken before he was born: "He saw a world that was practically unchanged—the same house, the same people—and then realized that he did not exist there at all and that nobody mourned his absence . . . what particularly frightened him was the sight of a brand-new baby carriage standing there on the porch, with the smug encroaching air of a coffin; even that was empty, as if, in the reverse course of events, his very bones had disintegrated."

Many years ago I sat in a cold French cathedral at a memorial mass for the deceased sister of my French composition teacher, listening to the priest talk about "LIFE"—about our lives and what we planned to do with them—and felt something akin to this. "This world doesn't need any of us," I thought. I felt as if we all were facing a wall of stone, that life itself was stone and we were buried in it. The somber occasion, the drafty, venerable edifice with its vaulted ceiling, the powerful music, the priest's words stirred my old nighttime foreboding. It wasn't a coincidence that this wave of anxiety tumbled over me in a cathedral. Cathedrals are meant to unmoor us from our certainties.

Theologian Paul Tillich wrote: "Anxiety is the self-awareness of the finite self as finite." Elsewhere he put it that anxiety is "finitude in awareness." This is anxiety with a capital A, not an anxiety we can hope to ever contain.

In an interesting essay on the French psychoanalyst and

thinker Jacques Lacan, Marshall Alcorn wrote that to Lacan anxiety is not a "defense" at all, but rather the very foundation upon which we erect our fragile sense of self. Thus it is not that anxiety conceals a truth (as Freud suggested), but rather that lying beneath the constructs we use to create a sense of order, control, and selfhood, anxiety *is* the truth. "It is not that the structures of the mind generate anxiety; it is that anxiety generates the structures of the mind." To Lacan, anxiety is therefore the fear that the self will be unmasked as a falsehood. Or, to quote Tillich again, anxiety is the realization that "nonbeing is a part of one's own being."

Paradoxically, this very terror is also the foundation for courage. "The courage to be," wrote Tillich, "is rooted in the God who appears when God has disappeared in the anxiety of doubt." As the religious Kierkegaard put it, anxiety is the doorway to another level of existence.

The deeper dreads will always be with us, and must be, I suppose. For them we need coping mechanisms of a different kind. Perhaps facing into the harsh wind of those ultimates does us the same kind of good that accepting the more local kind of panic, when it comes, can do. But when this ultimate dread informs our more trivial fears and problems, it is, in a sense, misplaced and unhelpful.

Justifiable fear is indispensable. Without fear we would have no concern for the future of the air, the oceans, our fellow creatures. Without fear nuclear war would have already incinerated the earth. Without fear there would probably be no art or love. Without fear we would not make wise choices in any domain.

It is possible that fear's unruly cousin and mimic phobia will also turn out to be useful. Perhaps its utility lies in its power to inhibit some common activities and thereby focus expertise on others of equal, if more obscure, value. Or like the feelings of confusion that occur during a panic attack—feelings that have in themselves no obvious usefulness but are the by-products of processes that do—the phenomenon of phobias, on the species level, may simply be an inconvenient by-product of a kind of sensitivity that the species urgently needs. Just as cells take on different roles in an organism, so the different types of human attributes emphasized in different people may prove advantageous to the larger organism of *Homo sapiens*.

I can't help wondering if as humankind has essentially stabilized, we haven't continued to diversify in minute ways in order to create a habitable human ecosystem. As in the evolution of the horse from little *Eohippus,* small differentiations must be continuing to express themselves in individuals, some of them bringing with them deleterious side effects, even though the essential evolution of our species has leveled off. The species must continue to need diversity in order to survive and flourish, and the growth of the new always occurs at a faster rate than the dwindling of the obsolete.

Perhaps people like me are like the browsers, the early horses that fed on softer leaves, gradually becoming extinct, while the grazers, which fed on hard grasses, survived. The browsers survived for millions of years, even after they had reached a kind of obsolescence in relation to their environment.

The development of the horse's stable, springy hooves also went through numerous distinct phases. As late as the last ice age there were still many protohorses with three toes on each foot, each of them with hooves. Perhaps phobias are the equivalent of the two side toes, which helped stabilize the central hoof, like training wheels on a child's bicycle, and survived in some strains of grazers for several million years. These side toes, though now obsolete, diminished slowly, almost as if they were watching to make sure that the horses could truly stand and run without them.

In that case neurotic anxieties would be no more than endowments from ancient times that have outlived their utility. Do we really need to run and hide when we hear a clap of thunder? Is this not, at this point in evolution, a mistake, the psychic equivalent of lower back pain, the result of nature's slow winnowing of defects?

Or is an unusual level of anxiety and caution in fact a valuable form of differentiation? As humanity continues to seek survival, might it not be finding increasingly subtle ways to satisfy its needs, including the need for meaning, for beauty, for complex thought, for metaphorical expression? I prefer to believe that certain types of neuroticism are the inevitable accompaniments of characteristics that nourish the human organism as a whole. So multifarious is existence that infinite varieties of attention are required to build a sustainable life within it. Those who particularly notice what is worrisome or anticipate—even to their detriment—what will be painful may be just those who notice nuances of life others might neglect. A species in which everyone was General Patton would not succeed, any more than would a race in which everyone was Vincent van Gogh. I prefer to think that the planet needs athletes, philosophers, sex symbols, painters, scientists; it needs the warmhearted, the hardhearted, the coldhearted, and the weakhearted. It needs those who can devote their lives to studying how many droplets of water are secreted by the salivary glands of dogs under which circumstances, and it needs those who can capture the passing impression of cherry blossoms in a fourteen-syllable poem or devote twenty-five pages to the dissection of a small boy's feelings as he lies in bed in the dark waiting for his mother to kiss him good night. It needs people who can design air conditioners, and it needs people who can inspire joy.

Phobias are widespread, but they still bear the dual stigma of being both "psychological" problems and not, statistically, "normal." In the minds of many, they demonstrate a failure of will and a flaw of character. If they are someday determined to be an entirely chemical or biological problem, attributable to a genetic defect like that which causes the peanut allergy, perhaps they will lose their stigma.

We are gradually working our way toward a new definition of psychology. The field we used to think of as somehow pertaining only to "the mind" now, finally, describes the intersection of mental life, experience, behavior, genetics, neurology, physiology, and evolution.

The concept of normality is also overdue for an overhaul. "Normality" is a relative term. Normality "floats." Each human being is a peculiar balance of assets and defects, physical, psychological, sociological. When you see a person's strengths, they are, by and large, eclipsing equally powerful weaknesses. Indeed the presence of outstanding strengths presupposes that energy needed in other areas has been channeled away from them. We should not be surprised to find some variety of mental anguish inside even the most "normal" exterior; we should assume it. People are infinitely layered. There are those who are sturdier in a crisis and bear up well under life's assaults. We need such role models before us to steady us on our way. And to aspire to a sense of balance in the face of life's challenges is certainly sensible. But those same sturdy people may fail in important spheres. So often does one discover serious deficiencies in those who superficially seem to function well, and compensatory strengths in those who appear to function less well, that it is tempting to suggest a more flexible model of mental health than that which we rely upon for convenience. In those who are remarkable for their sangfroid and equanimity, whose shadows do not show, just where are the darker forces that animate all nature but that only man has the ability to conceal? They may be buried deep, only to reemerge in actions with dire consequences. In the end, whatever people achieve that is most wonderful, beautiful, interesting, and inspiring is, by definition, not normal. And the corollary of this fact is that great achievements tend to come at a cost. Perhaps our best hope is to add something positive to the world and to do no great harm through our defects.

To be sure, we shouldn't be complacent about our weaknesses and should push ourselves to be useful, healthy, and fully alive. But there is no one template for a full life.

There is much to genuinely fear, and it is part of our uniqueness as creatures that we know this. But there are also unnecessary fears that get in our way and are well worth overcoming. Surely first and foremost of the fears worth dispensing with is the fear of letting others know our authentic selves.

But were we to neutralize our suffering and inner turmoil, would we not also lose our capacity to feel things deeply and to exult? As Friedrich Nietzsche wrote, "One must still have chaos in oneself to give birth to a dancing star."

This morning I was lying in the bathtub and I drifted into a mood of benign calm. It is winter, and the blanket of snow outside my window muffled the outer world. I could hear the sound of the water running in the pipes and the faucet dripping occasionally in a softly resonant plop, but it was so quiet I could almost imagine that I was outside time, a creature awaiting birth. I stared absently at the bare walls; I sensed my own body, but dimly, as if it were floating in space, without, in a sense, my noticing anything about it. I started to think about how much we need to keep our perceptions of external reality, which could so easily be overwhelming, in some kind of hierarchy. How strange it is that calm entails a kind of even attention directed to the body as a whole, with nothing in particular attracting interest. And how strange that my sense of being myself, a small creature in a tub of water, is in the foreground, with my awareness of the four white walls of the bathroom slightly receding into the background. And beyond that perception, in diminishing perspective, is a consciousness of the world directly outside the window, and then the world beyond that, and the world beyond that, and the immensities, the dark immensities beyond all these worlds. But those immensities are too far away and too big to be grasped. The imagination perceives them squintingly, trying, but failing, to bring them into focus. It is strange, we begin to really perceive these immensities in moments of ecstasy, or listening to music, when the world seems to open up again and again until there is no end to it. And at such times these endless spaces may be the greatest solace we have. And in moments when we are seized by terror we also feel the immensity of things erupting, as if inside us, to tell us that we are part of something vast and incomprehensible. At these moments we are most connected with all that is.

Acknowledgments

I could never have written this book without the support, insight, and expertise of family, friends and colleagues, nor without the research and eloquence of the many authors whose works I studied in preparation for writing it. In the Selected Readings section I have listed some of the books I found particularly indispensable in my attempt to understand the psychological, physiological, and evolutionary underpinnings of phobia. I would particularly like to acknowledge the helpfulness of Charles Darwin's *Expressions of the Emotions of Man and Animals*, David Barlow's *Anxiety and Its Disorders*, Maryanne Garbowsky's *The House Without the Door*, and Reinhold Heller's *Edvard Munch: The Scream*.

I want to extend my deepest thanks to Dr. Marjorie LaRowe, Dr. Patricia Miller, and to Dr. Stephen Reibel, without whom the content of this book would have been immeasurably poorer, if indeed it could have existed at all. To my friend Frederick Seidel, I send a special thank-you for his suggestions and support. I am deeply indebted to those family and close friends who have offered me encouragement and advice during the period of writing, many of whom read the manuscript at various stages along the way; these include my children, Annie Shawn and Harold Shawn, my brother Wallace Shawn, Deborah Eisenberg, Jill Fox, Kathleen Tolan, and Maria Guida. I want to thank Yoshiko Sato, owner of Kiwi, for her insight, forbearance, companionship, and the warm encouragement she gave me throughout the process of planning and writing this book. Among other colleagues, friends, and experts who offered invaluable help, guidance, and support, I particularly wish to thank Henry Chapin, Anda Constantine, Dr. Jane Danien, Priscilla Gilman, Jay Hamburger, Ben Harvey, Deborah Mills Hayes, Amy Hotch, Suzanne Jones, Pamela Lawton, Charles McGrath, Christopher Miller, Neil Moss, Piergiorggio Nicholetti, Dr. Mark Reber, Linda Smith, and Oceana Wilson.

I am enormously grateful to my agent Lynn Nesbit, for her helpfulness, and to my editors Wendy Wolf and Hilary Redmon, for their support, patience, guidance, and virtuosic editorial skills. In addition I wish to extend great thanks to Carol Cott Gross and to Dr. Frederick Stern for their willingness to talk with me and for sharing their knowledge. I owe a particular debt of gratitude to my colleagues at Bennington College whose words are cited in this book, and who were so generous with their time and support and suggestions throughout this project: Dr. Ronald Cohen, Dr. Elizabeth (Betsy) Sherman, Dr. Bruce Weber, Dr. Kerry Woods, and student Michelle Hogle (who is currently pursuing a Ph.D. in neuroscience at Boston University). During those times while writing this work when its unifocal self-description began to remind me unpleasantly of Nikolai Gogol's story "The Nose," in which a civil servant awakens to find that a giant version of his own nose has gotten dressed, put on a coat, gone to work, and assumed a life of its own, their brilliance and interest in the topic as something of general usefulness cheered me and inspired me to press on with it.

Selected Readings

Andreasen, Nancy C. *The Broken Brain*. New York: Harper Perennial, 1984.

Barlow, David H. *Anxiety and Its Disorders*, 2nd ed. New York: The Guilford Press, 2002.

Barlow, David H., and Michelle G. Craske. *Mastery of Your Anxiety and Panic*. San Antonio, TX: Harcourt Brace, 1994.

Bettelheim, Bruno. *Freud and Man's Soul*. New York: Vintage Books, 1987.

Breuer, Joseph, and Sigmund Freud. Nicola Luckhurst, trans. *Studies in Hysteria*. London: Penguin Books, 2004.

Brown, Janet. *Charles Darwin: vol. I: Voyaging, vol. II: The Power of Place*. London: Jonathan Cape, 1995, 2002.

Cannon, Walter B. *The Wisdom of the Body*. New York: W. W. Norton and Company, 1963.

Carter, Rita. *Mapping the Mind*. Berkley: University of California Press, 1999.

Damasio, Antonio. *The Feeling of What Happens*. Orlando, FL: Harcourt, Brace, 1999.

————. *Searching for Spinoza*. Orlando, FL: Harcourt, Brace, 2003.

Darwin, Charles. *The Expression of the Emotions in Man and Animals*. New York: The Philosophical Library, 1955.

Daves, Graham C. L., ed. *Phobias: A Handbook of Theory, Research and Treatment*. West Sussex, UK: John Wiley and Sons, 1997.

Dickinson, Emily. *Final Harvest*. Boston: Little, Brown and Company, 1961.

Dobzhansky, Theodosius, Francisco J. Ayala, G. Ledyard Stebbins, and James W. Valentine. *Evolution*. San Francisco: W. H. Freeman and Company, 1977.

Eysenck, H. J. *Sense and Nonsense in Psychology*. Bungay, UK: Penguin Books, 1957.

Freud, Sigmund. David McLintock, trans. *The Uncanny*. London: Penguin Books, 2003.

————. James Strachey, trans. *Symptoms and Anxiety*. London: W. W. Norton and Company, 1959.

————. James Strackey, trans. *The Complete Psychological Works. vols. III, VII*. London: The Hogarth Press, 1997.

————. *Three Case Histories*. New York: Touchstone Books, 1963.

Garbowsky, Maryanne M. *The House Without the Door*, London: Associated University Presses, 1989.

Goleman, Daniel. *Emotional Intelligence*. New York: Bantam Books, 1995.

Goodwin, Donald W. *Phobia: The Facts*. Oxford: Oxford University Press, 1983.

Grandin, Temple. *Emergence*. New York: Time Warner Books, 1986.

————. *Thinking in Pictures.* New York: Vintage Books, 1996.

Halgin, Richard P., and Susan Krauss Whitbourne. *Abnormal Psychology.* Orlando, FL: Harcourt Brace Jovanovich, 1993.

Hallowell, Edward M. *Worry.* New York: Ballantine Books, 1997.

Heller, Reinhold. *Edvard Munch: The Scream.* New York: Viking Press, 1972.

Huxley, Julian. *Evolution in Action.* New York: Penguin Books, 1968.

Kierkegaard, Søren. Reider Thomte, trans. *The Concept of Anxiety.* Princeton: Princeton University Press, 1980.

Marks, Isaac M. *Phobias and Rituals.* New York: Oxford University Press, 1987.

————. *Fears and Phobias.* New York: Academic Press, 1969.

Melville, Jay. *Phobias and Obsessions.* Middlesex, UK: Penguin Books, 1977.

Pascal, Blaise. *Pascal's Pensees.* New York: E.P. Dutton, 1958.

Pavlov, I. P. G. V. Anrep, trans. *Conditional Reflexes.* Oxford: Oxford University Press, 1927.

Rachman, S. *Phobias: Their Nature and Control.* Springfield, IL: Charles C. Thomas, 1968.

Rachman, Stanley, and Padma deSilva. *Panic Disorder: The Facts.* Oxford: Oxford University Press, 2004.

Roazen, Paul. *Freud and His Followers.* New York: Alfred A. Knopf, 1976.

Sacks, Oliver. *An Anthropologist on Mars.* New York: Vintage Books, 1995.

Saul, Helen. *Phobias.* New York: Arcade Publishers, 2001.

Schmidt, Leonard J., and Brooke Warner, eds. *Panic: Origins, Insight and Treatment.* Berkeley, CA: North Atlantic Books, 2002.

Stoodley, Bartlett. *The Concepts of Sigmund Freud.* Glenooe, IL: The Free Press, 1959.

Sulloway, Frank. *Freud: Biologist of the Mind.* New York: Basic Books, 1983.

Vander, Arthur, James Sherman, and Dorothy Luciano. *Human Physiology.* New York: McGraw-Hill, 2001.

Willheim, Richard, ed. *Freud: A Collection of Essays.* Garden City: Anchor Books, 1974.

Wullschlager, Jackie. *Hans Christian Andersen.* New York: Alfred A. Knopf, 2001.

Zane, Manuel D., and Harry Milt. *Your Phobia.* New York: Warner Books, 1984.

Index